Soak an Egg in Vinegar
  —for a calcium-rich eggnog, shell and all

Drink "Hard" Water
  —it may keep you from a heart attack

Try Brewer's Yeast
  —for a full ration of zinc, chromium and phosphorus

Chew a Clove of Garlic
  —for the selenium which allows full benefit
    from protein

These may seem like old wives' folk remedies—yet each
provides minerals needed for the body to function.

In this up-to-date comprehensive guide to the little-un-
derstood role of minerals in human nutrition, Dr. Carl
C. Pfeiffer, noted head of the Brain Bio Center in
Princeton, New Jersey, explains how health, disease and
life itself, are influenced by the mysterious effects of
those minerals that make up so vital a part of our diet—
and of our bodies.

Dr. Carl C. Pfeiffer's
UPDATED FACT/BOOK ON

Zinc and Other Micro-Nutrients

Keats Publishing, Inc.　　　　New Canaan, Connecticut

Some of the material in this book
originally appeared in
Mental and Elemental Nutrients
by Carl C. Pfeiffer, Ph.D., M.D.

ZINC AND OTHER MICRO-NUTRIENTS
Pivot Original Health Edition published 1978

Library of Congress Catalog Card Number: 77-91327
PIVOT ORIGINAL HEALTH BOOKS are published by
Keats Publishing, Inc.
36 Grove Street
New Canaan, Connecticut   06840

ACKNOWLEDGEMENTS

The author is indebted to Eric Braverman for help in preparation of this book. The excellent typing of both Marie Arcaro and Phyllis Loften is deeply appreciated. The author also acknowledges the many patients who gave of their blood and urine to partially untangle the snarl of the schizophrenias. The original data presented in this book are based in part on the work of our laboratory crew directed by Arthur Sohler, Ph.D. and Rhoda Papaioannou, M.S.

CONTENTS

FOREWORD

THE ASTUTE CLINICIANS know that excessive thirst in a pale patient may indicate internal bleeding. The body is alerted by the decreased blood volume to drink water. Similarly, the dog with nausea and diarrhea will eat grass to replenish the body's supply of potassium and magnesium—both salts are lost in the watery bowel movements. Adrenal deficient animals crave salty water and cats made neurotic by constant stress crave 10% ethyl alcohol—a drink which the normal cat would not even use for grooming.

Pica, the craving for non-edible unnatural "food" such as chalk, ashes, or clay, occurs in man and is nature's response to a profound mineral deficiency. The word pica (in zoology) is the genus which contains the European crow, the Magpie, a bird noted for the stealing of trivial food.

Pregnant women who are zinc deficient will eat clay or plaster with vinegar in an attempt to rectify the deficiency. This hidden hunger for minerals may motivate children to taste and swallow sundry objects which the adults abhor either because of the lack of nutritive content or the constant risk of poisoning. Such a child, aged 5, came under my care recently. The pica responded completely to modern mineral (micro-nutrient) therapy.

Carol was brought to my office on January 5, 1976.

Her mother described the problem which developed as soon as the baby was able to put things into her mouth and she began eating non-edible things. She tried to explain this to her pediatrician and he said that all babies put things in their mouths and she replied "but she just doesn't put things in her mouth, she eats them and swallows them." He retorted with the usual statement which pediatricians make: "she'll outgrow it!" The mother went on to relate that when Carol was still in the creeping stage she loved to lick the top of the Comet cleanser can and licked like she was really enjoying it. As she grew her appetite increased and included other non-edibles such as candles which she "literally devoured." Although she became very sick from eating candles she returned again and again to this "forbidden fruit." She ate crayons of all colors, chalk and even ate the graphite out of pencils. She fancied all cosmetics, particularly lipsticks, and ate them down to the bottom of the container. When she played outdoors during the pleasant weather, she ate spoonfuls of dirt and sand with the expressions of joy a normal child makes when eating ice cream. She would eat rather than play with "Silly Putty" or "Play Dough." To this, she added matches, cigarettes and papers of all kinds. She swallowed everything she chewed.

A mineral analysis done on Carol's hair revealed below normal levels of potassium, cobalt, manganese and zinc. Her magnesium, copper, iron and lead were all considerably above normal. Lead level was 29 parts per million (normal—6 to 12 ppm). Carol's treatment was started with niacinamide, pyridoxine, vitamin C, vitamin B-12, manganese citrate, zinc gluconate, folic acid, all administered twice daily; and sodium alginate, a natural substance made of seaweed and used to remove heavy metals from the body, once daily. On her return visit in March 1976, her parents reported that between four to six weeks after starting the vitamins and minerals, Carol began to awaken announcing to her mother that she was hungry and wanted to eat. For the first time in her short life, she was asking for food and her mother added that the only non-edible which Carol had consumed in these past weeks was one chopstick.

They returned with Carol on May 2, 1977, and reported that Carol was a totally different child. Her shyness had receded and physically she had made marked changes. Her hair is glossier, has better texture, doesn't break off as it used to, her skin color is better and her cheeks are rosy. Learning improved although she went through a four month period when she was having letter and word reversals which had now receded.

A repeat hair analysis dated April 14, 1977, revealed the following:

Copper had been reduced to 3 ppm; iron to 18 ppm; and lead had been reduced from 29 ppm to 8 ppm which is well within average range. Manganese increased from less than 1.0 ppm to 0.5. Zinc rose from 135 ppm to 184 ppm. The ease with which these results can be obtained never ceases to amaze me.

Modern society provides a perfect salt lick rich in minerals for the farm animals. The salt cake is no longer white but rather solid pink minerals mixed with the yellow elemental sulfur. Perhaps we need such a salt lick for the crawling infant.

This book on zinc and other micro-nutrients should be in the hands of every mother, nurse and teacher, all of whom deal with the normal development of infants and children.

ALLAN COTT, M.D.

CHAPTER 1

Zinc as an Essential Element

DURING these days when the cloudy viewpoint of the FDA limits the clinical investigation of DMSO (dimethylsulfoxide) because massive doses in the dog produce lens cloudiness, we recall the eye-opening history of an antituberculosis drug named ethambutol (Myambutol Lederle). This drug represents a solid chemotherapeutic advancement but, even more, a genuine triumph for man over animals in the realm of chronic toxicity.

The Question of Testing in Man

In 1960, an international gathering of clinical pharmacologists assembled in the Midwest to discuss the amount and type of animal data needed before trials in man could be started on a new candidate drug. Some were ultraconservative and wanted extensive animal studies, and some wisely stated that almost everything should be carefully tried in man since animal studies can only give guidelines as to biochemical systems which might be blocked or damaged in man.

To test the faith of the liberals, Dr. Paget (then with the Imperial Chemical Industries in Britain) stated that he had made extensive chronic toxicity studies of an effective chemotherapeutic agent against tuberculosis but that, unfortunately, it produced blindness in three dif-

1

ferent species of animals at the high dosage used in the chronic toxicity studies. Could this be tested in man?

Most looked at him incredulously, but some of us had faith in man's biochemically unique structure and suggested cautious trial in a few patients with slowly increasing dosage—if permission could be obtained from the local drug committee and the patient volunteers.

What helped some of us to keep the faith were faint but distinct memories of a time when we charted eye grounds weekly in patients receiving tryparsamide therapy for their neurosyphilis. Some may also have recalled that extremely large doses of quinine (tonic water) can reduce human vision by action on the retina.

Quite independent of the British study, a division of the American Cyanamid Company, Lederle Laboratories, had developed a drug which they knew to be a chelater of zinc ions and which was also highly effective in tuberculosis. In the dog, chronic toxicity testing disclosed that the drug at high dosage produced a pallor of the *tapetum lucidum* (iridescent layer of choroid of the eye). This is the membrane in the back of the eye that is responsible for the bright reflections (eye shine) from animal eyes when it is activated by automobile headlights. This membrane acts as a photomultiplier to allow animals to see better in the dark. The fluorescent reaction depends on an adequate supply of zinc-containing enzymes, so that the pallor produced by the candidate drug was understandable and on a sound scientific basis. The zinc was chelated and partially removed. Human and other primate eyes do not have a *tapetum lucidum;* therefore, cautious clinical trial in tuberculosis patients was started, and the drug was found to be highly effective.

In the meantime, chronic toxicity testing in the cat disclosed retinal detachment at the high dosage used. The highest level of zinc in the human brain occurs in that extension of the brain which is the retina of the eye. Thus, zinc is also important in the visual process in man.

As a trace metal, zinc is important in biochemical processes of tissues other than the retina. Therefore, great reassurance was supplied by Dr. Buyske and his colleagues at Lederle when they completed their dog and monkey studies which showed that the trapping or chelation of zinc by ethambutol was much greater for the eye than for the pancreas, heart or liver. The clinical trials still went forward cautiously, with careful attention being paid to the vision and ophthalmoscopic (eye) findings in each patient.

With all these warnings from the faithful laboratory animals, imagine the dismay of the clinical investigator when he discovered on morning rounds a tuberculosis patient who appeared to be reading the newspaper upside down! The patient admitted he had not been able to read newspaper print for several days. The drug was discontinued and the patient's vision soon returned to normal. At a later date, reinstitution of ethambutol therapy at a lower dose was not accompanied by any reduction of visual acuity.

The patient's explanation for pretending to have normal vision was simple—and a real moral lesson. He had been hospitalized for more than five years with tuberculosis and had not responded to surgical or standard drug treatments for his tuberculosis. In spite of the best available medical care, he saw himself going out the back door of the hospital as had many of his friends. He, personally, chose to go out the front door—even if he went out blind! This is a logical choice for anyone to make.

Dr. I. D. Bobrowitz of New York City, one of the pioneer clinical investigators of ethambutol, stated in 1966 in the *Annals of the New York Academy of Sciences:*

> There was not a single instance of definite eye toxicity due to ethambutol (i.e., complaints of poor vision, poor color discrimination, decrease in visual fields, and scotomas.) There were many patients on our study in whom there were fluctuations in reading of the Snellen eye chart with a reading loss or improve-

ment. These variations occurred with similar frequency in all regimens, with or without ethambutol.

At the same New York Academy of Sciences Symposium, Drs. Donamae and Yamamoto, of Japan, reported that they had found side-effects in only 22 out of 187 patients treated with ethambutol. The drug was stopped in only 5. In 3 cases the drug was discontinued because of a decrease in visual acuity which later returned to normal.

The drug package insert that accompanies Myambutol gives careful directions for the evaluation of eye changes and the need for constant testing of vision, as with the now historic tryparsamide chemotherapy.

The critical and authoritative *Medical Letter,* in its 31 May 1968 issue, states: "With the doses now recommended, reported ocular effects have generally been minor and reversible, though one consultant has noted some permanent loss of visual acuity due to ethambutol in two patients."

The drug has been acclaimed by Dr. Gordon Meade, Director of Medical Education for the American Thoracic Society, as "An excellent drug . . . that will probably be widely used." The drug is particularly beneficial when used with the previous antituberculosis drugs to prevent the development of drug-resistant strains.

Ethambutol still can produce blindness in many species of lower animals, but thanks to the ability and patience of the pharmacologists, pathologists and clinical investigators at the Lederle Laboratories, the drug has been assayed in man and found to be useful in the treatment of one of man's oldest maladies—tuberculosis.

This human-interest saga reinforces the statement made repeatedly by Bernard B. Brodie that new drugs must be tested in man as well as in animals. We must not let animal studies or governmental committees, either local or national, interfere with the continued fight against crippling diseases. Perhaps this ethambutol report may help to get DMSO out of its present limbo.

Since the whole human populace is borderline-deficient in zinc, these side actions of ethambutol might be lessened if each tuberculous patient were given a dose of zinc and vitamin B-6 at a time interval spaced away from the ethambutol therapy. In the early days, many schizophrenic patients succumbed to tuberculosis and many more had chronic tuberculosis. In one Illinois state hospital the percentage of tuberculous mental patients was 6.5. Early investigators postulated that a toxin from the tubercle bacillus might cause schizophrenic symptoms, since the patient who got well from his tuberculosis also got well from his schizophrenia.

Perhaps the good nutrition therapy of the past, including foods containing zinc, may be the common denominator in the treatment of both diseases. With soil depletion of zinc and other essential elements, the old-fashioned nutrient-and-rest therapy for tuberculosis might not be effective today. Fortunately, we now have specific antituberculosis drugs.

Discovery of Zinc as an Essential Element   The Wisconsin group of biochemists who carefully determined in 1928 that copper was needed concluded from animal experiments by 1934 that zinc was an essential element also. They concluded that man needed zinc, but E. J. Underwood of the Institute of Agriculture University of Western Australia in 1962 stated in *Trace Elements of Human and Animal Nutrition* that zinc deficiency had never been observed in man. However, a skin disease of pigs, reported in 1955 by Tucker and Salmon, was found to be a zinc deficiency, and at about that time animal feeds were supplemented, since O'Dell and Savage had shown that chickens also needed extra zinc for maximal growth. Some feeds and dog foods are supplemented to the extent of 200 ppm of zinc as soluble salts. This extra zinc has increased feed efficiency up to 25 percent in swine and poultry and is one of the reasons for the comparatively low cost of pork and chicken in the United States.

The American *human* diet contains only one-tenth that of animal feed, namely 15 to 25 ppm of zinc. Soil exhaustion, food processing, careless cooking and the consumption of junk foods all contribute to this low level. Man should get 15 mg of zinc per day, but analyses of well-rounded diets served at cafeterias and hospitals show that only 8 to 11 mg of zinc per day is provided. Institutional diets are even lower in their total available zinc content.

Lack of Zinc in Soils   Since zinc, like iodine, sulfur, and selenium, occurs in the soil as water-soluble salts, excessive rainfall can leach the zinc from the soil. Glaciated areas (e.g., many northern sections of the United States) may have soils deficient in zinc. This is well known to agriculturists who advise the addition of zinc to fertilizers. In Florida, where the sandy soil has little in the way of trace elements, zinc is a routine metal in fertilizer. Some land plants accumulate from the soil as much as 16 percent of their ashed weight as zinc. When a crop containing 100 ppm of zinc is removed from a field, the soil will lose 1 ppm of zinc. The best soil contains only 50 ppm of zinc, so theoretically 50 such annual crops would exhaust the soil in fifty years or two generations. Some of the fertile lands of the earth have been tilled for many centuries and their zinc content is totally exhausted. Such soils occur in Egypt, Iran and Iraq, where the first zinc-deficient humans were found.

Dwarfism, Hypogonads and Failure of Sexual Maturity   In 1961, Prasad, Prasad and Halstead published a detailed clinical study of eleven Iranian male dwarfs who, in addition to iron deficiency, had, by modern tests, zinc deficiency. The symptoms were dwarfism at the age of twenty years, infantile sex organs and lack of mental acuity. The iron deficiency was corrected without improvement. Later, in a controlled study on seventeen male dwarfs, the control group of eight on a normal diet required 224 days for normal sexual activity, while the nine fed the normal diet plus 100 mg of zinc sulfate each day developed normal sexual function in 59 days—4 times as fast. These twenty-year-old dwarfs grew in height because the growing ends of the long bones had not closed. The hospital diet produced 4.2 cm of increased height, while the same diet plus zinc produced 10.5 cm—more than twice as much.

The normal diet of the Iranian villages from which these patients came consisted in large part of unleavened bread which contains phytate, a compound that prevents the absorption of zinc. (In the cities of Iran leavened [yeast-raised] bread is used.) We now know that the biochemical process of leavening bread destroys the phytate.

What Factors Modify Our Zinc Intake? At present no factor *increases* our zinc intake. In the "olden days," the use of galvanized (zinc-coated) food-processing vessels resulted in some useful zinc contamination. Now stainless steel is used instead. In the case of water pipes, acid well water took off some of the lining of the galvanized pipes and provided zinc (but also some cadmium because the zinc was not pure). Now acid drinking water gives us too much copper.

Many factors *decrease* the effective zinc in food and water in modern society. If the plant, grain, fruit or nut has enough zinc from the soil, then it will have a normal zinc level. In the case of lettuce, we know that farmers can grow great greenery without the requisite zinc and manganese if they just put lime and nitrate on the soil. With *adequate* fertilization and scientific farming, the zinc should be there for the eating!

Scientific farming differs from organic farming in that the available trace elements such as zinc are determined and the fertilizer adjusted to fit soil conditions. Organic farming may (as in Europe) add the manure of animals that have been fed 250 ppm of copper in their food. Manure from animals with this amount of copper can poison the soil of the unsuspecting organic farmer! The easiest type of scientific farming is hydroponics, wherein only diluted minerals—and no soil— are used. Sprouting of seeds for food approaches scientific farming.

Food Processing Removes Zinc Food processing is designed, however, to remove anything from food that will discolor, turn rancid or attract bugs. Bugs cannot grow without zinc, so 80 percent of the zinc is removed from wheat flour in the milling process. Cornstarch has much less zinc than corn meal. Frozen peas have less zinc than backyard peas because the surface layer of trace metals is removed with EDTA to produce a brighter green when the peas are cooked. This can happen to broccoli and spinach too. This bright green may be more appealing but is certainly less nutritious.

In the preparation of foods, the vegetable pot liquor may go down the drain, taking the water-soluble zinc salts with it. (But if not thrown away, the water used to cook vegetables may be high in copper from the copper plumbing or pan bottom, and copper antagonizes zinc in the body.) Red meat is a good source of zinc, but the hamburger may contain the cheaper protein from the soybean which is high in copper and low in zinc. The frankfurter may be loaded with cereal which, with its phytate content, will prevent the absorption of any zinc which wanders in with the meat. The oyster is commendably high in zinc, and 100 gm of Atlantic oysters will provide 120 mg of zinc— enough for a whole week if the body could only store zinc. However, along with the zinc in the oyster there occurs copper in large amounts and cadmium in great excess if the oyster is grown in contaminated waters. This makes the oyster less desirable as a source of zinc. Under the best circumstances, the level of zinc in any modern diet may be minimal, contaminated or downright missing. Hence the need for zinc supplements.

Levels of Zinc in Man All told, Bartlett's *Familiar Quotations* list 101 separate items on gold. Silver merits 39 items and *zinc is not even listed.* Yet, to the body, zinc is more precious than gold. This is "Truth purer than the purest gold."

While rodents and nocturnal animals have higher levels of zinc in the back of the eye (retina), man in general has higher tissue levels of zinc than animals. If we except the retina and pineal gland in the brain, the highest level of zinc in the brain is in the hippocampus, where histamine is also present.

Several studies have been made on trace metals in the brain. Harrison et al. in 1968 studied copper, zinc, iron and magnesium distribution in the human brain. They found copper to be highest in the caudate nucleus, zinc and magnesium highest in the hippocampus and iron highest in the globus pallidus. Ibata and Otauka, in 1969, using histochemical techniques, found zinc to be present mainly in the terminal vesicles of the nerve endings of the hippocampal formation of rabbits and rats. The zinc was distributed as follows: hippocampus, 95 ± 38 mcg per gm; caudate, 81 ± 21; putamen, 75 ± 13; globus pallidus, 69 ± 16; corpus callosum, 49 ± 30; thalamus, 58 ± 9. Thus, of the parts of the brain tested, the hippocampus has the highest zinc level.

Since zinc occurs with histamine in both basophils and mast cells, one can speculate that the terminal vesicles of the mossy fibers of the hippocampus may be histaminergic—that is, a nerve impulse may be generated when histamine is released.

Histamine: Neurotransmitter Stored with Zinc

Histamine is a biochemical which normally occurs in all soft tissues of the body. It is made by the removal of the acid group from the amino acid histidine. This amino acid can apparently be made in the bodies of adults but perhaps not in those of children. Histidine is usually not listed with the essential amino acids. Both histamine and histidine will chelate, or nab onto, trace elements such as copper and zinc. Perhaps because of this, histidine is available as a food supplement and is occasionally used in the treatment of arthritis. We know that one factor in arthritis is a tissue overload of copper, iron or other heavy metals—thus, the chelating action of extra histidine is beneficial in that these metals are removed from the body.

Swedish scientists have studied histaminergic nerves for many years, and others have noted that histamine will increase stomach acid secretion and salivary secretion. Histamine may therefore be a humoral agent which will be released in the brain and cause the transmission of neuronal impulses. Dr. Michaelson of Cincinnati was the first to use the ultracentrifuge to separate the rat brain into particles of various sizes to test for the presence of histamine in the small vesicles which carry the neurotransmitters in the brain cells. He found histamine in this vesicle fraction, and his work has been confirmed by Kataoka and De Robertis of Buenos Aires and also by Snyder and Taylor of Baltimore.

All of these workers have studied the subcellular localization of histamine in rat brain, using the same separation methods that have been used to demonstrate the presence in synaptic vesicles of the other brain transmitters acetylcholine, norepinephrine, dopamine and serotonin. When the mitochondrial and microsomal-20 fractions are disrupted, a high concentration of histamine is found in these vesicle subfractions. The presence of histamine in small nerve endings and in synaptic vesicles of rat brain cortex suggests a transmitter role for histamine as well as for the other biogenic amines. In other words, histamine is a neurotransmitter in some as yet unspecified portion of the brain.

Several workers have studied the hippocampal mossy fibers for their zinc content; others have studied these same areas of the brain for histamine content. These studies are doubly important in that these may be histaminergic fibers, and the hippocampus is an important structure in regard to integration of thoughts, memory and emotions. If the histamine, of the histaminergic nerve fibers, is stored with zinc, as histamine appears to be in both the mast cell and the basophil, then a functional role of histamine storage could be ascribed to the zinc in the terminal vesicles of the mossy fibers.

The use of zinc in the storage of the neurotransmitter histamine of the hippocampus has been suggested in 1971 by Niklowitz. Haug et al., in the same year, found that the depletion of zinc in the hippocampus after degeneration of the mossy fibers is compatible with the concept of a neurotransmitter role for zinc. McLardy, in 1973, found a decrease in the cells of the hippocampus in both schizophrenics and alcoholics. Any deficiency in mossy fiber cells, or of zinc or histamine in the cells, might result in schizophrenic behavior.

Other Signs of Zinc Deficiency While the original studies on zinc deficiency in males disclosed infantile sex organs, dwarfism and anemia, we know that many more signs and symptoms of zinc deficiency can be detected by the informed clinical observer.

Skin The skin may show striae (stretch marks) over the hips, thighs, abdomen, breasts and shoulder girdle. Young ladies present themselves with mental difficulties and with striae of the skin to such an extent that they cannot wear a bikini. Young men who have tried to exercise away their disperceptions by weight lifting present themselves with striae in the skin of the shoulder girdle. As one lad put it, "I was in a YMCA class in weight lifting and I was the only one out of twenty-five who developed stretch marks. I could feel my skin breaking as I lifted the weights." His initial blood serum level of zinc was 60 mcg percent, compared to a normal of 100 mcg percent. Hair and nails do not grow well and the brittle nails may have white spots or be generally, opaquely white in zinc deficiency. The hair will be brittle and lack pigment, and may change to a deeper color with zinc therapy. We have seen carrot-red hair turn auburn and dead-white hair turn to a rich brown. The facial skin may have acanthosis, a severe form of acne; the skin lesions frequently clear with zinc and vitamin B-6 therapy.

Sex and Endocrine Problems The zinc-deficient girl may not have a regularly established menstrual cycle until age fourteen to seventeen, or the menses may start at thirteen, only to skip for months or even a year. If treated with birth control pills (to regularize the cycle) the patient will have a rise in serum copper which may precipitate depression and intensify disperceptions. However, if placed on vitamin B-6 and zinc, these patients usually establish a normal menstrual cycle within two to three months. Since normal ovulation may start first, it is even possible for a young lady who is at risk (if she is not using effective contraceptive measures) to become pregnant before she menstruates.

With impotent young males who are zinc deficient, a return of sex function may take as long as four to five months of daily zinc supplementation. They may sometimes have an abnormal fear of microphallus (small penis), but with zinc and vitamin B-6 the sex organs develop to full size and the beard and axillary hair become more abundant. Masturbation or sex become more gratifying.

Joint Pain Painful knee and hip joints may plague the teen-ager who has zinc deficiency. One such patient had such painful knees that he chose rowing in prep school because he knew he could not run. We know that poultry with zinc or manganese deficiency get hock disease. We know that active children in the eight-to-thirteen-year-old period are subject to interruption of the blood supply of the growing head of long bones (Perthes' and Osgood-Schlatters' diseases). The zinc-deficient patient has cold extremities with poor peripheral circulation. Because of previously acquired needle trauma, these patients may dread having to give a blood sample. Frequently we must warm the hand and arm before blood can be obtained. They may faint with blood sampling. As they become less zinc-deficient, blood taking is no longer an ordeal; furthermore, they no longer faint. With poor circulation and this tendency to faint, the zinc-deficient patient is a poor risk for dental anesthesia and other operations. Care should be taken to recognize the zinc-deficient patient and correct the deficiency before elective operations. Not only will the patient be prone to shock, but bleeding can be abnormal and wound healing will be delayed.

Retarded Wound Healing Drs. Walter Pories and William Strain have pioneered in the careful study of wound healing in zinc-deficient patients. Most surgeons give salt, glucose and sterile water to their patients in the postoperative period; some surgeons realize that the alcoholic needs more magnesium and vitamins; some surgeons use Ringer's solution which contains the chlorides of sodium, potassium, calcium and magnesium. Some surgeons prepare their patients for operation by assessing nutrient status and give them preoperatively what their patient lacks. Drs. Pories and Strain use zinc salts preoperatively and postoperatively to promote wound healing and to correct zinc deficiency.

Stress of any kind depletes the body of zinc—so much so that the burned patient ends up with body tissue zinc at such low levels that normal healing is retarded. Some of these patients have serum zinc levels of 30 mcg percent (one-third of normal). Most burn centers now use dietary zinc supplements in all their patients, many of whom are young and need all the zinc they can get for normal growth. Burns are so painful that the stress causes great losses of zinc via the urinary pathway and also in the exuding of fluid from the burned area.

Loss of Taste Several side actions of chelating agents should have suggested that one of the vital trace metals was involved in the sense of taste. When penicillamine was introduced for the treatment of Wilson's disease (excess copper) the side-effect of loss of taste occurred as the excess copper was removed from the body. But chelating agents (and penicillamine is no exception) are seldom specific for a given metal. With penicillamine, copper and zinc are both removed and the zinc must be replaced or side actions such as loss of taste occur.

After publishing his finding that copper, nickel and

zinc were involved in loss of taste, Dr. Robert I. Henkin finally settled on zinc deficiency as the main factor in hypogeusia (loss of taste). Older patients, particularly those with cancer, are particularly prone to this annoying symptom. When the mother has loss of taste, she oversalts all the food served to the family. When loss of smell and taste occur, the usual early recognition that food is burning or the house is on fire must depend on other members of the family or other senses such as the visual detection of smoke or flame.

Dr. Henkin and his colleagues (for no good reason in our opinion) are against correcting the loss of taste with the most common salt, zinc sulfate. Numerous studies have shown that zinc sulfate is as well absorbed as other zinc salts, and chelated zinc has no special virtues. Dr. Henkin has not recognized that many patients with loss of taste are also deficient in vitamin B-6 (pyridoxine). (Zinc will not work without other nutrients, including vitamin B-6.) In our clinical experience, patients with loss of taste should be given B-6 for the first two days. Otherwise, zinc alone can increase hallucinatory experiences and/or depression. Patients with loss of taste are usually severely depressed, and for a good reason: the food they eat tastes like so much sawdust.

Birth Defects The nauseated pregnant woman is usually deficient in both vitamin B-6 and zinc. Both are needed for growing tissues of any kind, and the fetus in the uterus makes extraordinary demands on the mother's supplies. Vitamin B-6 has been used for nausea and vomiting of pregnancy with uneven success. We have had many pregnant patients who had difficulty with previous pregnancies go through a pregnancy on a zinc and B-6 nutrient program with no difficulties.

Several workers, notably Dr. Lucille Hurley of the University of California, have shown that zinc deficiency in pregnant rats will result in many stillborn pups and that those born may have one of a number of birth defects. Dr. Caldwell and his colleagues in De-

troit have shown that the rats born of zinc-deficient
mothers are mentally retarded and do not learn as well
as rats born to zinc-supplemented mothers. Our colleagues visiting Iran and Egypt are told that 30 percent
of the young children are slow learners. These areas of
the world no longer have available zinc in much of the
soil.

TABLE 1.1

Clinical disorders and possible zinc deficiency

Syndrome	Associated B-6 deficiency	Scientist	Place
Dwarfism	+	A. Prasad	Iran
Poor growth	+	Hambidge	U.S.A.
Hypogonadism	+	Prasad	Iran
Hypogonadism	+	Caggiano et al.	U.S.A.
Wound healing	?	W. Pories	U.S.A.
Loss of taste and smell	?	R. I. Henkin	U.S.A.
Cadmium poisoning	?	H. A. Schroeder	U.S.A.
Cirrhosis of liver	+	Sullivan et al.	U.S.A.
Parenteral nutrition	+	M. E. Shils	U.S.A.
Poor circulation	?	J. H. Henzel	U.S.A.
Childhood hyperactivity	+	Allan Cott	U.S.A.
Epilepsy	+	A. Barbeau	Canada
Diabetes	+	E. J. Underwood	Australia
Enlarged prostate	?	I. M. Bush et al.	U.S.A.
High cholesterol	?	H. G. Petering	U.S.A.
Effects of oral contraceptives	+	R. Alfin-Stater	England
Psoriasis	?	Voorhees et al.	U.S.A.
Cutaneous striae	+	Pfeiffer et al.	U.S.A.
Pregnancy, nausea	+	Pfeiffer et al.	U.S.A.
Kwashiorkor	?	S. Kumar and K. S. Jaya-Rao	India
Acanthosis	+	Hallbook	Sweden
Acrodermatitis enteropathica	+	E. J. Moynahan	England
Acne	+	Pfeiffer et al.	U.S.A.
Sickle cell disease	?	S. Dash et al.	U.S.A.
Lack of ovulation	+	Pfeiffer et al.	U.S.A.
Impotency & amenorrhea	+	Pfeiffer et al.	U.S.A.

Syndrome	Associated B-6 deficiency	Scientist	Place
Coarse hairs— eyebrows	?	F. M. Dementzis	Greece
Body and breath odor	?	F. M. Dementzis	Greece
Pyroluria, white spots in nails, lack of dream recall, disperceptions, hallucinations, or depression	+	Pfeiffer et al.	U.S.A.
Retinal detachment	+	Pfeiffer (postulated)	U.S.A.
Reye's syndrome	?	Pfeiffer (postulated)	U.S.A.

Male Growth Lag Have you ever attended an eighth-grade dance and seen tall girls dancing with boys who only came up to the girls' shoulders? In contrast, at the junior prom or twelfth-grade dance, you see girls only coming up to the boys' shoulders. Why do the boys lag in growth behind the girls? One does not see this disparity in growth between the two sexes in the animal kingdom, where most pet foods are over-adequate in their supply of zinc. Gaines dog food, for instance, has a zinc content which is a hundred times the recommended level. Male pups do not lag behind the females in growth as they become sexually mature.

The sex organs of boys are loaded with zinc in their mature or functioning state. During puberty, as the prostate, seminal vesicles and testes develop, the body's borderline zinc supply is taxed severely to provide all the zinc needed for the male sex glands to function. To compensate, the voracious appetite of the growing male teen-ager finally overcomes this hypothetical, but probably real, zinc deficiency in the four-year period from eighth to twelfth grade.

Since junk foods and soft drinks contain no zinc, the growing teen-ager who consumes them needs, more than ever, his whole grains, eggs, milk, vegetables and meat. We know from the Iranian male dwarfs that short stature and hypogonadism can result from zinc deficiency. Parents should make sure that this does not happen to their son, since failure to develop sexually can lead to many neuroses.

Summary In summary, then, the situations in which zinc deficiency or copper excess may occur are:

1. During pregnancy, when growth and development require zinc.
2. During the first year, when the newborn has excess copper and needs zinc to balance the copper.
3. During rapid growth, the child requires adequate zinc.
4. From the twelfth year, zinc is required for normal pubertal development of the male, and deficiency may cause a growth lag. The pubertal development of the female may require less zinc.
5. During the teen-age years, at the time when zinc is lowest and copper is high, premenstrual tension occurs. This is an endocrine effect which might be corrected with additional dietary zinc.
6. From fifteen to twenty years, stress of any kind causes loss of zinc, and in some people stress causes the excretion in the urine of kryptopyrrole, which takes with it both zinc and vitamin B-6.
7. In adult life, chronic zinc and B-6 deficiency may predispose cells to cancerous change. Wounds and burns require zinc to heal. Hypertensives are high in copper and low in zinc.
8. In older patients who suffer from confusion resulting in senile behavior, the confusion may be caused by excess copper.

Stretch Marks in the Skin (Striae) Clinicians have known that the stretched skin of the abdomen of the pregnant woman may break under the surface layer and leave scars. This also happens in some obese individuals. Surprisingly, many women go through several pregnancies without any stretch marks. This indicates that nutritional or familial factors may be involved. We see many young people with stretch marks in the skin owing to normal growth at puberty. The skin of the breasts, abdomen, thighs and hips is frequently scarred with these subcutaneous breaks. These breaks in the connective tissue also occur in diabetics and in persons who have excess cortisone secretion.

The two major components of connective tissue are collagen fibers and elastic fibers. The collagen fiber is formed by fibroblasts in the healing of wounds; the elastin is formed outside the cell in a manner similar to the manufacture of our modern polymers. Elastin is built rapidly and perfectly during normal growth, and the elastic fiber lives as long as the individual. Elastin comes from four molecules of lysine in a process fur-thered by lysyl oxidase—a copper-containing enyzme. This enzyme requires pyridoxal phosphate (vitamin B-6) to make either collagen or elastin fibrils (very small muscle fibers found in striated muscles). Vitamin C is also necessary in this process to stabilize the easily oxidized chemical groups of a metallo enzyme (enzyme containing a metal, such as a copper-containing enzyme). Both zinc and copper are needed for effective cross-linking of the elastin chains to make the perfect elastic tissue. When imperfect, any overstretching will cause long tears which appear as striae or stretch-marks.

Copper-deficient animals lack pigment in their hair and die of ruptured elastin in their main arteries. Zinc-deficient animals have hock disease—imperfect formation of cartilages—and cannot make B-6 phosphate. Animals deficient in B-6 would also lack skin and hair pigment, since B-6 phosphate is needed in the formation of both elastin and collagen. The biochemical cause of the stretch marks in teen-agers with pyroluria is thus understandable, because both vitamin B-6 and zinc are lost from the body in abnormal amounts.

Fingernail White Spots: Possible Zinc Deficiency
Many children and teen-agers and a few adults have white spots in the fingernails. These occur more frequently in the nails of the index and little finger of the dominant hand—i.e., the right hand for right-handed

individuals. Trauma is thus a factor, but not the primary cause, since patients with numerous white nail spots will also have such spots in the toenails. White banding may occur in the nails of both hands.

Attention was called to these spots or paired bands by R. C. Muerhcke in 1956. He ascribed the phenomenon to a serum albumin level lower than 2.2 gm per 100 ml. His largest group of patients suffered from nephrosis, and those in a second group had hepatic cirrhosis. All had low serum albumin levels. Two patients responded to cortisone therapy with disappearance of the white banding, and several patients responded to albumin-replacement therapy. We now find that spots or paired bands will occur in patients with zinc and pyridoxine deficiency that is metabolically induced by the abnormal excretion of kryptopyrrole derivatives which combine chemically with pyridoxal phosphate and then complex with zinc. These patients have normal serum protein levels but are zinc and pyridoxine deficient. The major portion (70 percent) of the serum zinc is bound to albumin and our observations are therefore in accord with Muerhcke's findings, since patients with albuminuria also have a significant zincuria and patients with hepatic cirrhosis have a very low serum zinc level.

Our suggestion is that the metabolic white banding of finger and toenails is primarily the result of zinc deficiency. This deficiency can be caused by zinc loss due to albuminuria as well as in other ways. We further find that with therapy, only small white spots resolve; large white spots must grow out with the fingernail, a process taking five to six months. The banding of the nails may result from the menstrual cycle in the female. Copper level is high and zinc is low one week before the menstrual period when women are more liable to depressive disorders.

Religious days of fasting may cause white spots that can be traced to the food abstinence in orthodox Jews, some of whom, like some of the rest of the populace, are borderline deficient in zinc.

An acute psychotic episode may be accompanied by

the broad white banding. Fasting with inadequate intake of zinc may accompany the psychosis.

The minimal daily requirement for zinc is 15 mg, but analysis of various diets shows an average of only 11 mg. Zinc deficiency may be aggravated by the ingestion of excess copper, as in drinking water or in vitamins plus minerals, many of which contain 2 mg of copper in each tablet. The situation can also be aggravated by increased estrogen ingestion—for example, in contraceptive pills. Pfeiffer and Iliev reported in 1972 that estrogens raise ceruloplasmin and serum copper and lower serum zinc.

Fingernail furrows known since 1846 as Beau's lines are crosswise depressions in the nail produced by a fever lasting a week or more. These furrows grow out with the nail so that the approximate date of the severe fever can be estimated by the slow forward march of the furrow, which takes one month to appear. The growth of the adult fingernail is 0.104 to 0.108 mm per day. The entire nail is replaced in 5½ to six months, but women with long nails may provide the doctor with almost a year of nail growth to inspect. (Once polish is removed!)

Women's nails are more brittle than men's. When men go on estrogens their nails become brittle within six months. The birth control pill makes women's nails more brittle. Brittle or thin nails are not helped by gelatin therapy. Nails are made stronger by zinc and sulfur supplements to the diet. The zinc can be in the form of zinc gluconate tablets, and the sulfur is most conveniently given as eggs (yolks). The diet should, of course, contain adequate protein.

Dermatologists have named these white spots *leukonychia*. Some internists have stated (without giving evidence) that these spots are deposits of calcium. The more frequent occurrence of these spots in teen-agers than in atherosclerotic patients is evidence against the calcium hypothesis. Actual analysis shows no increase in calcium, but the zinc level rises, as does the copper level.

The types of white spots are summarized below (see Figure 1.1).

1. Frequent small white spots in the nails of people living in historically glaciated countries. (Glaciers leached iodine, sulphate, selenium and zinc from the soil.)

2. Fasting or "Yom Kippur" white spots. (The whole populace is so borderline deficient in zinc that one to two days of fasting may produce white spots.)

3. Menstrual white bands. (Serum zinc is low at the menstrual period, while serum copper is high. This results in rhythmic monthly banding, since six months are required for the nail to be replaced.)

4. Weekly or fortnightly bands produced by dietary binges.

5. White bands seen in backpackers, perhaps because of zinc lost in sweat and also because of their frequent avoidance of red meat in their backpacked diet.

6. Influenza white spots, with a furrow in the nail if the patient had a high fever at the time of the influenza. (If the patient is not zinc deficient, only the furrow occurs. Pecarek and Biesel have shown that most types of virus infections deplete the body of zinc.)

7. "We ran out of zinc" white spots. (Teen-aged patients will develop white spots if they fail to take their zinc dietary supplement over a weekend or if they run out of zinc before the next visit to the physician.)

8. A homogeneous white opacity in the entire nail, instead of white spots. (When adequate zinc and vitamin B-6 are given, sections of the nail corresponding to the months in which this therapy took place have a normal pink appearance.)

9. After treatment with zinc, the opaque part of the nail grows out and is replaced by normal healthy pink nail.

Miller Laboratories of West Chicago, Illinois, markets a Zn-Plus which contains 5 mg of zinc combined with soy protein and torula yeast. For most people this dose of zinc would be too low, and the company has not proven that better absorption of zinc occurs with their product. Several studies have shown

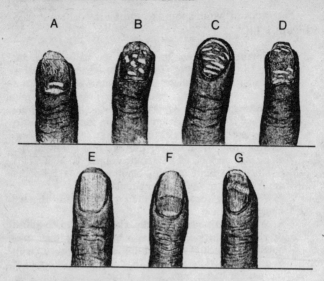

Types of white spots on fingernails (leukonychia) seen in zinc-deficient patients

A. Isolated white spot originating from a period of fasting or altered diet. Yom Kippur fasting, or a day of anorexia can cause such a white spot. A back-packing trip (which usually does not include fresh red meat as a source of zinc) can also produce a white spot. A hospital stay of 5 days also caused a white spot indicating the low level of zinc in that hospital's diet.

B. Multiple white spots in the finger and toe nails of an eleven-year-old child whose serum zinc level was low and whose behavior was inappropriate.

C. Monthly white bands or menstrual white spots in a female pyroluric patient. Copper is high and zinc is low premenstrually when many women feel depressed.

D. White spots in the nail of a female pyroluric patient who ran out of zinc and vitamin B-6 after a 2½ month period of treatment. The center band of normal-appearing nail represents the period of zinc therapy.

E. Opaquely white nail of an older pyroluric patient who also had hypertension and elevated serum copper. The hypertension rsponds to zinc and vitamin B-6 therapy and the nail becomes normal pink in color.

F. Opaquely white nail after 3 months of zinc B-6 therapy.

G. White spot in a depression in the nail (Beau's Grove) caused by a virus infection with a high fever. Virus infections cause a loss of zinc via the urinary pathway and the altered metabolic rate of a fever results in the transverse groove.

that zinc as the sulfate is adequately absorbed. The other PDR (1974) preparations of zinc are too low to be useful.

Plus Products have a Formula 85 which contains 15 mg of zinc as the gluconate plus unstated amounts of manganese and magnesium in a mixture of bone meal and dolomite. The price is competitive with that of zinc gluconate tablets.

For use by children, most pharmacists, on a doctor's order, will make up a 10 percent solution of zinc sulfate which can be used three drops morning and night. This dose provides 5 mg of zinc in soluble form, which for a child would approximate half of the needed daily intake.

Zinc is like many other trace metals: the body will ordinarily take from the intestines only the daily needed amount; the rest will not be absorbed. An exception might be metallic zinc in an oily base, since an Iranian youth became oversleepy when he ingested zinc and peanut butter.

What Doses of Zinc Are Safe?   In the latest edition of the *U.S. Pharmacopoeia* zinc sulfate is listed as a substance to be used orally as an emetic. For a while a midwestern company that markets zinc sulfate $7H_2O$ in pellets of 220 mg could not ship its product to the many surgeons interested in wound healing without a label reading, "Dissolve 4 tablets in water and use as an emetic"! This peculiarity of bureaucracy is a hint as to the safety factors of the soluble salts of zinc. If too much is taken, then vomiting will occur. The patient who slowly takes increasing amounts of zinc will probably develop diarrhea before he has nausea and vomiting. Either of these symptoms requires a decrease in dosage.

As with most trace metal salts, only a certain percentage of the swallowed zinc dose will be absorbed from the stomach and intestine. An excess may lead to nausea and diarrhea. In the case of iron, we are only modestly protected and children can easily be poisoned by eating a bottle of candy-coated iron salt tablets. The same may be true of soluble zinc salts if they are ever (God forbid!) supplied in the form of candy-coated pills. Even the dose forms presently available should be kept out of the hands of children.

As Dr. Murphy reported in the *Journal of the American Medical Association* in 1970, a lad of sixteen living in Tehran, Iran, read in *Time* magazine for 19 November 1965 that zinc was good for wound healing. He had a minor wound, and he had just purchased 12 gm of elemental zinc to use as a rocket fuel. He therefore mixed the zinc with peanut butter, spread it on his bread, and ate it all to speed his recovery. The next day he had difficulty awakening and staying awake at breakfast. He also fell asleep in school. The sleepiness increased over the next four days and on the fifth day he was taken to the U.S. Air Force hospital in Tehran for treatment.

On the morning of admission he was difficult to arouse, but when awakened he consumed a normal breakfast and then returned to sleep while sitting on a stool. He was dizzy, staggered as he walked, and wrote illegibly. He had no nausea and denied any diarrhea. Reflexes and speech were normal, and he successfully completed simple psychological tests. Many laboratory tests were done, and the only abnormalities were slightly high activities of serum lipase and amylase. He recovered the next day and a follow-up a month later disclosed no abnormality. On the eighth and fifteenth days after dosing, his serum zinc level was not abnormally high.

We know that ingestion of alcohol with fat will delay absorption of the mixture, so the slow release of zinc from the peanut butter might be expected. It is surprising that this rash act did not result in greater harm. As a matter of fact, if this procedure could ever be proven safe, many insomniacs would consider zinc and peanut butter a real blessing. The elemental zinc must have been of high purity; otherwise the lad would have ended up with cadmium or lead poisoning. Both of these substances are more poisonous than zinc.

The most recent scientific study on the safety of zinc

in man was done by Czerwinski et al. in Oklahoma in 1974. To sixteen geriatric patients these doctors administered 220 mg zinc sulfate three times a day, which is a large dose for patients in their sixties. Diarrhea occurred in six of the sixteen patients. In four weeks plasma zinc rose from a normal average of 100 mcg percent to 150 mcg percent and remained at this high level for the twenty-four week duration of the study. Some behavioral tests indicated that several of the zinc-treated patients might have benefited. The urinary, blood, kidney and liver tests did not differ from the findings in the fourteen patients who, as controls, received placebo capsules. From this and other studies we can state that this large dose of zinc as the sulfate is probably very safe.

Most patients do not need 220 mg doses, particularly when zinc is given with B-6 and E vitamins. The one exception may be those patients with psoriasis. Vorhees et al. found in 1969 that these patients need more than the usual zinc dietary supplement.

The elevation of serum zinc from a normal of 100 mcg percent to 150 mcg percent might seem dangerous. If more B-6 were given the rise might have been less. However, we have many patients who are deficient in B-6 and live for months with serum zinc levels of 150 to 300 mcg percent. These levels fall to the 100 to 150 mcg percent range when adequate B-6 is given. These patients may have an increase in their abnormal mental symptoms if zinc dietary supplementation is started before the B-6 deficiency has been treated. In epileptics, seizures may increase unless the B-6 therapy is started first.

In summary, we have treated over 1,700 patients with zinc dietary supplements, using various salts, and have not seen a serious side-effect attributable to the zinc alone. The use of a double dietary supplement such as zinc and manganese in a ratio of twenty to one can raise blood pressure. This is helpful in the hypoglycemic, but in the older patient the blood pressure level must be monitored at regular intervals.

Case History: Fran and the Fried Oysters Before listing the food sources of zinc, we must summarize the case history of Fran, a baby adopted at the age of two weeks in August 1955. Although Fran was overactive as a baby, her parents saw no evidence of difficulty until she started school, where she repeated the first grade because of poor learning.

Her behavior and learning problems seemed to be emotional in nature, but psychological counseling did not help. In the sixth grade she was diagnosed by a psychiatrist as having minimal brain dysfunction and later by a clinic as having learning disabilities involving poor visual perception and auditory memory.

At age thirteen her pediatrician, believing her erratic and irritable behavior might be caused by low blood sugar, finally hospitalized her for three weeks and placed her on a high-protein, sugar-free diet plus vita-

TABLE 1.2

Dietary supplements of zinc, magnesium and manganese in the physicians' desk reference (PDR)

Manufacturer *(sells to pharmacies)*	*Pharmacist* *(sells to the public)*
Meyer Laboratories, 1900 W. Commercial Blvd., Ft. Lauderdale, FL 33309.	Willner Chemists, 330 Lexington Avenue, New York City, NY 10016.

Vicon-C		*Zimag-C*
Ascorbic acid	300 mg	is the same as Vicon-C.
Nicotinamide	100 mg	
Magnesium sulfate, USP (As 50 mg dried magnesium sulfate)	70 mg	
Zinc sulfate, USP (As 50 mg dried zinc sulfate)	79 mg	
Thiamine mononitrate	20 mg	
D-calcium pantothenate	20 mg	
Riboflavin	10 mg	
Pyridoxine	5 mg	

Vicon Plus

is the same as the above
with 4 mg of manganous
chloride added.

Ziman Fortified

is the same as Vicon Plus.

Supplements

Health food stores now have in stock zinc tablets (as the gluconate) in various sizes. The 15 mg content of zinc is the
most popular since this represents the daily needed intake of
zinc metal for each adult.

---

mins. After she had been in the hospital a few days her
behavior—which had been extremely antagonistic and
uncooperative much of the time—dramatically and
suddenly changed. The unprovoked temper tantrums
involving ranting and raving, the cruel swear words—
all suddenly stopped.

The parents tried to keep her on a sugar-free diet at
home. However, for a less-than-cooperative teen-ager
this was almost impossible, especially since she seemed
to have a craving for candy. They learned, after repeated experiences, that candy or candy wrappers
could usually be found in her room after one of her
destructive tantrums. However, she still was in much
better condition than before they knew about the
sugar. She still was immature, had very poor logic,
made mostly C's and D's in school. But the tantrums
had decreased in frequency and in degree.

Her parents had noticed several years before that after Fran had eaten fried oysters she was always unusu-
ally alert and cooperative—and never had any
tantrums. So they all ate fried oysters an awful lot.
They kept wondering what could be in the oysters that
could have this effect on her. The parents' massive
reading program included the book *Orthomolecular
Psychiatry,* in one chapter of which Pfeiffer describes a
high-histamine-level patient in a way that seemed to fit
Fran and recommended a zinc dietary supplement.
They also found, in a book on nutrition by Roger
Williams, that oysters contained 143 mg percent of
zinc and that the next best source of zinc was roast

beef, with only 6.4 mg percent zinc. This had to be the answer!

Although the parents had tried megavitamin therapy without any significant improvement, they had again started Fran in August 1973 on a closely supervised megavitamin dosage of mostly vitamin C, niacinamide (2 to 3 gm daily) and B-6. After four months of this therapy, they could not ascertain any significant improvement. Then, on 27 December 1973, they gave her the first dose of zinc. The very next day she was positively improved. Within two weeks after she had started the zinc she had (1) obtained her driver's license (for two years she had had a learner's permit but had not wanted to try for the license); (2) obtained a full-time job from midnight to 8 A.M. (the first job she had ever had); and (3) enrolled in a college for a three-hour-per-day course (she had been out of high school for several weeks and had not previously expressed any desire to attend college). Although after two more weeks she had to drop the college—no time for sleep—they just couldn't believe the change that had taken place in their Fran.

They continued the megavitamins for two months and gave her one Vicon Plus (Meyer Lab multivitamin with 80 mg zinc and 4 mg manganese) in the morning and one chelated zinc (Rich-Life, Inc., 200 mg zinc) in the evening. Then, they stopped the megavitamins completely (except what was in the Vicon Plus) but continued the zinc. There was no discernible change— the very great improvement remained. They continued the zinc for a total of 3½ months (from 27 December), then stopped everything to see what would happen. For two days there was little change, but on the third day Fran had a "blowup"—a real temper tantrum. The next day, another. This one included the ranting alone in her room. It was the first time such ranting had taken place since she had begun receiving the zinc. One week after they stopped the zinc her behavior had deteriorated so much that they felt they had to resume it. They gave her the zinc capsule at 8:30 A.M.; by

6:00 that night she was, once again, a changed person—and continues to be, as the zinc is continued.

Fran still has problems. She is immature, still has poor logic (although this seems to be improving) and few friends. Her parents have a strong feeling that she has lost the sugar compulsion, although they are not yet certain. But after eighteen years of watching Fran try to cope with her frustrations and failures, the parents thank God she is not in prison. No one can imagine how much the parents are enjoying the new Fran. They say, "She has a great sense of humor, is considerate and fun to be around. *There is no doubt whatsoever in our minds that zinc has saved her.*"

Zinc Responsive Disorders in Farm Animals

For more than fifty years, New Zealand agriculturalists have sought effective means of preventing and treating a fatal disease which afflicts farm animals in this country during the autumn. The disease, caused by a fungus toxin found in certain pasture grasses, produces liver damage and severe facial eczema (abnormal sunburn) in sheep and cattle. It has cost New Zealand farmers millions of dollars in deaths, damage to stock livers and lower production.

Recent studies, based on the observations of Mrs. Gladys M. Reid, a New Zealand dairy farmer, indicate that zinc sulfate is an effective prophylactic for the disease. Mrs. Reid has long been concerned over the numbers of New Zealand breeding stock that develop difficulties late in pregnancy. Extreme muscular weakness, a teetering walk, failure to eat enough and gain weight, eczema on the face and at the base of the tail, failure to lift the tail with subsequent soiling and lethargy precalving are symptoms of what New Zealand farmers term "the sulky cow syndrome." If the animal does not collapse in the last week of pregnancy, she will produce a dead or weak calf after prolonged and stressful labor.

Mrs. Reid found that animals who suffer this condition could be revived by coaxing them to eat hay

TABLE 1.3

Food sources of zinc

Mg per 100 gm = 3 oz

Vegetables*		Sea foods	
Peas	4.0	Atlantic oysters	143
Carrots	2.0	Herrings	100
Beets	0.93	Hard clams	21
Cabbage	0.80	Soft clams	21
Watercress	0.56		
Asparagus	0.32	Meats	
Rutabaga	0.30		
Lettuce	0.30	Pork liver	9.0
Potato	0.29	Beef liver	5.5
Corn	0.25	Lamb	5.3
Tomato	0.24	Beef	6.4
Sweet potato	0.23	Chicken thigh	2.8
Cauliflower	0.23	Chicken breast	1.1
Green beans	0.21		
Turnip greens	0.21	Cereals*	
Turnips	0.08		
		Wheat bran	14.0
Fruits*		Whole oatmeal	14.0
		Wheat germ	13.3
Dates	0.34	Whole corn	2.5
Banana	0.28	Unpolished rice	1.5
Pineapple	0.26	White rice	0.5
Red currants	0.20		
Lemon	0.17	Breads	
Prune juice	0.16		
Cherries	0.15	Whole rye	1.34
Apricots	0.12	Whole wheat	1.04
Orange juice	0.11	White	0.12
Grapefruit juice	0.10		
Cantaloupe	0.09	Dairy products†	
Pears	0.08		
Peaches	0.07	Whole egg	1.5
Apple juice	0.07	Egg yolk	1.5
		Egg white	0.02
Nuts*		"Egg Beaters"	0.46
		Cow's milk	17-66
Whole nuts	3.42	Human milk	2-138
Peanut butter	2.0	Human colostrum	70-900†

* Actual level in food crops depends on adequate zinc level in the soil. Many soils are deficient. In the case of cereals, the calcium phytate present in the products will prevent the absorption of zinc. Thus, the available zinc may be less. The

soaked in molasses and a special proprietary stock meal, both extremely high in zinc.

Mrs. Reid was familiar with the studies of Dr. Jean Apgar of the U.S. Agricultural Research Service which showed that zinc deficient laboratory animals suffer considerable lethargy in advanced pregnancy and have a long and difficult labor. She began administering zinc sulfate to her "sulky cows." Given one teaspoon (about 5 grams) of zinc sulfate "straight down the throat" even the most seriously ill animals ("downer cows") were on their feet within hours, their appetites returned in several days and they gave birth to healthy calves.

Zinc is stored in the liver and Mrs. Reid observed that the collapse of the cow with toxin-induced liver damage occurred at the same time, and in a similar manner, to the collapse of the zinc deficient animal at the birth of the young. In fact, most of the "sulky cows" were professionally diagnosed as suffering from previous liver damage.

Mrs. Reid's observations interested scientists of the Ruakura Agricultural Research Center near Hamilton, New Zealand. In laboratory studies, these scientists found that rats fed synthetic diets deficient in zinc became severely ill and died shortly after admininstration of the fungus toxin while rats fed synthetic diets supplemented with zinc escaped serious liver damage when

feeding of copper to chickens and pigs (a practice which is legal at 250 ppm of copper in England and Europe) results in high copper and low zinc levels in the liver. These livers frequently end up in liver sausage which may be inedible because of the high copper content. Foods or drinking water high in copper can negate much of the zinc obtained from food.

† The human infant is born loaded with copper. This can be corrected by an adequate zinc intake. Notice that human colostrum (first breast secretion) is high but variable in zinc content, perhaps for this specific purpose. But note also that the variability of human milk is from *2 to 138* mg percent, while the better-fed cows have a variability in the zinc content of their milk from only *17 to 66* mcg percent. Rather than on milk from a zinc-deficient mother, the baby might thrive better on cow's milk. The obvious answer is to give the mother zinc.

the fungus toxin was administered and survived. In field trials, using sheep and milking cows, large doses of oral zinc sulfate significantly reduced toxin-induced liver damage following administration of the fungus toxin. Scientists conclude that oral zinc sulfate, in large doses, will protect farm animals against the fungus toxin.

In another study, New Zealand veterinarian, Dr. B. F. Rickard, divided a group of 50 yearling calves affected with facial eczema into two mobs. Twenty-five calves were treated with oral zinc sulfate while the remaining calves served as controls. Within 10 days, the treated group showed considerable improvement. The animals' skin lesions were healing well, they gained weight and their coats began to shine. Animals in the control group failed to improve and many died.

These studies confirm Mrs. Reid's observation that zinc sulfate is the key to solving the animals' health problem which has long troubled New Zealand farmers.

Mrs. Reid has also found zinc supplementation beneficial for improving the health and disposition of young animals. Weaning is a stressful situation for the little calves. Separated from their mothers, the calves refuse to eat, crowd together and bellow constantly. When she recalled that Dr. Apgar had found zinc to be stress-protective, Mrs. Reid put zinc sulfate in the weanlings' watering troughs. The following day the young animals were peacefully grazing and were spread all over the paddock.

Mrs. Reid further notes that when calves are fed extra zinc they are happy and play. She comments that, "in a large herd, the younger animals are pretty low on the social order. After a few days on zinc sulfate, the calves kick their heels in a frisky fashion. They walk in a purposeful way and their tails are not soiled because they lift their tails high to defecate in a purposeful way."

Mrs. Reid's experiences indicate that the addition of zinc salts to farm watering troughs could contribute greatly to the prevention of disease states and the promotion of optimal health in farm animals.

References

Apgar, J. Effect of zinc repletion late in gestation on parturition in the zinc deficient rat. *Journal of Nutrition* 103: July 1973.

Bush, I. M.; Sadoughi, N.; Shah, M. S. and Berman, E. Zinc: a key urological element. Presented at the meeting of the American Urological Association, Washington, D.C., 1972.

Caldwell, D. F. et al. *Proc. Soc. Exp. Biol. Med.* 133:1417, 1970.

Calhoun, N. R., Smith, J. C. and Becker, K. L. The role of zinc in bone metabolism. *Clinical Orthopedics.* 103:212–234, 1974.

Czerwinski, A. W.; Clark, M. L.; Serafetinides, E. A.; Perrier, C. and Huber, W. Safety and efficacy of zinc sulfate in geriatric patients. *Clinical Pharmacology and Therapeutics.* 15:436–441, 1974.

Dolar, S. G. and Keeney, D. R. Availability of Cu, Zn and Mn in soils. *Journal of Science Fd. Agriculture* 22:273–286, 1972.

Fernandez-Madrid, F., Prasad, A. S. and Oberleas, D. Effect of zinc deficiency on nucleic acids, collagen and non-collagenous protein of the connective tissue. *Journal of Laboratory and Clinical Medicine* 82:951–961, 1973.

Fjerdingstad, E., Danscher, G. and Ferdingstad, E. J. Zinc content in hippocampus and whole brain of normal rats. *Brain Research* 79:338–347, 1974.

Garbarg, M.; Babbin, G.; Feger, G. and Schwarz, J. C. Histaminergic pathway in rat brain evidenced by lesions of the medial forebrain bundle. *Science* 186:833–835, 1974.

Halstead, J. A., Smith, J. C. and Irwin, M. I. A conspectus of research on zinc requirements of man. *Journal of Nutrition* 104:345–378, 1974.

Hardjan, P. M.; Smith, C. G.; Herman, J. B. and Halstead, J. A. Serum zinc concentration in acute myocardial infarction. *Chest* 65:185–187, 1974.

Harrison, W. W., Netsky, M. G. and Brown, M. D. Trace elements in human brain: copper, zinc, iron and magnesium. *Clinica Chimica ACTH* 21:55–60, 1968.

Haug, F. M. et al. Timm's sulfide-silver reaction for zinc during experimental anterograde degeneration of hippocampal mossy fibers. *J. Comparative Neurology* 142:23–31, 1971.

——Depletion of metal in the rat hippocampal mossy fiber system by intravital chelation with dithizone. *Histochemie* 28:211–219, 1971.

Haug, F. M. On normal histochemistry of trace metals in the brain. Presented at the Trace Elements and Brain Function Symposium, Princeton, New Jersey, 1973.

Henkin, R. J. Zinc in wound healing. *New England Journal of Medicine* 291:665–674, 1974.

Hurley, L. S. The consequences of fetal impoverishment. *Nutrition Today* 3:2, 1968.

Hussey, H. H. Taste and smell deviations: importance of zinc. *JAMA* 228:1669–1670, 1974.

Ibata, Y. and Otsuka, N. Electron microscopic demonstration of zinc in hippocampus formation using Timm's sulfide-silver technique. *J. Histochem. Cytochem.* 17:171–175, 1969.

Kazimierczak, W. and Maslinski, C. Effect of zinc ions on selective and non-selective release in vitro. *Agents and Actions* 4:1, 1974.

McBean, L. D.; Dove, J. T.; Halstead, J. A., and Smith, J. C. Zinc concentrations in human tissues. *Amer. J. Clin. Nutr.* 25:672–676, 1972.

McClain, P. E.; Woley, E. R.; Beecher, G. R.; Anthony, W. L. and Hsu, J. G. Influence of zinc deficiency on synthesis and cross-linking of rat skin collagen. *Biochimica et Biophysica ACTA* 304:457–465, 1973.

McLardy, T. Hippocampal zinc and structural deficit in brain from schizophrenics and chronic alcoholics. Presented at the Trace Elements and Brain Function Symposium, Princeton, New Jersey, 1973.

Muerhcke, R. C. The fingernails in hypoalbuminuria: a new physical sign. *Br. Med. J.* 195:1327–1328, 1956.

Murphy, J. V. Intoxication following ingestion of elemental zinc. *JAMA* 212:2119–2120, 1970.

Niklowitz, W. J. Interference of Pb and Mg with essential brain tissue Cu, Fe and Zn as main determinant in experimental metal encephalopathy. Presented at the Trace Elements and Brain Function Symposium, Princeton, New Jersey, 1973.

O'Dell, B. L. and Savage, J. E. Effect of phytic acid on zinc availability. *Proc. Soc. Expt. Biol. Med.* 103:304, 1960.

Pecarek, R. S. and Biesel, W. R. *Appl. Microbiol.* 18:482, 1969.

Pfeiffer, C. C. and Iliev, V. A study of zinc deficiency and copper excess in the schizophrenias. *Int. Ref. Neurobiol.* Supp. 1:141–165, 1972.

Pories, W. J.; Henzel, J. H.; Rob, C. G. and Strain, W. H. Acceleration of wound healing with zinc sulfate. *Ann. Surg.* 165:432, 1967.
Pories, W. J. and Strain, W. H. Once upon a trace metal: the zinc story. *Medical Opinion,* 7, 1971.

Prasad, A. S. *Zinc metabolism.* Springfield, Illinois: Charles C. Thomas, 1966.

Reid, G. M. (Personal communications)

Rickard, B. F. Facial eczema: zinc responsiveness in dairy cattle. *New Zealand Veterinary Journal* 23:41–42, 1975.

Rodale, R. The zinc story. *Prevention,* July 1973.

Schroeder, H. A. Losses of vitamins and trace minerals resulting from processing and preservation of foods. *American Journal of Clinical Nutrition.* 24:562–573, 1971.

Strain, W. H., ed. *Clinical applications of zinc metabolism.* Springfield, Illinois: Charles C. Thomas, 1975.

Towers. Role of $Zn+^2$ in protecting against sporedesmin damage. Biochemistry section, Ruakura Agricultural Research Center, August 1975.

Tucker, H. F. and Salmon, W. D. Prakeratosis or zinc deficiency in pigs. *Proc. Soc. Expt. Biol. Med.* 88:613–616, 1955.

Vorhees, J. G.; Chakrabarti, S. G.; Botero, Fernando; Miedler, L. and Harrell, E. R. Zinc therapy and distribution in psoriasis. *Arch. Derm.* 100:669–673. 1969.

Zinc Toxicity Update 1978

ZINC is the least apt of the trace elements to produce toxic effects in man. Single large doses produce vomiting and diarrhea, while small continued doses are ordinarily absorbed only to that extent which meets the body's needs. At the onset of therapy, excess zinc can displace copper from the tissues, temporarily worsening psychiatric depression. Extra zinc in the intestine may hinder the absorption of iron. Early in zinc dietary supplementation, the individual may be less tolerant of alcohol, so that a single beer may produce sweating and dizziness. This occurs to a greater extent with Antabuse, a drug designed to stop the oxidation of alcohol at the aldehyde stage; with continued use of zinc this alcohol intolerance disappears. Patients on zinc sweat more but this is probably a good normal response to heat and emotion.

Can Continued Zinc Therapy Drive Copper or Iron Too Low?

Zinc supplements may increase serum copper for a period of two to three months, but with continued zinc and vitamin C the copper level decreases to a normal level. Zinc dietary supplements keep serum copper level at 90 to 100 mcg percent and zinc level at 120 to 140 mcg percent. In my opinion these are the ideal levels for maximal benefit in the prevention of disease. Repeated serum levels are more informative than repeated hair samples or the attempted estimation of copper and zinc in food or water intake.

Alice the Hyperactive Athlete In January 1974, a sixteen-year-old hyperactive girl, whom we shall call Alice, visited the Brain Bio Center. She was barely manageable because of lack of bladder control (day and night), eczema with constant scratching so as to produce bleeding, screaming, aggressive behavior—she frequently bit her parents—mental retardation and lack of speech but fair recognition of loud commands. Any stranger to her was Grandma or Grandpa! She had frequent left upper abdominal pain and constipation. Brain waves were reported normal, and neither Thorazine nor Stelazine was effective. She was then on Prolixin but with little benefit; when she would finally sleep, she would sleep too long and was difficult to awaken.

Examination of Alice at the Brain Bio Center revealed pyroluria (urinary kryptopyrrole 93 mcg percent) (normal 10), hypercupremia, serum copper 144 mcg percent (normal 100), which crested to 158 mcg percent on the second visit five weeks later. Two months later, on the third visit, the serum copper had come down to an almost normal 114 mcg percent and it stayed normal until September 1976. We will return to the copper story later.

Alice became a new person on zinc and B-6 therapy. Her skin eczema cleared in six weeks as did her constipation, bedwetting and stomach pains. She was able to sit and watch TV, and she began to use small phrases such as "I'm hungry," and "going to Princeton tomorrow." Her menstrual period became regular and her bladder control was perfect both night and day. Alice still had her ups and downs and occasionally needed 50 to 75 mgm of Thorazine at bedtime for sleep.

Finally, at age eighteen, in the spring of 1976, Alice was, in her parents' words, 98 percent better but still overactive. She was now a good swimmer and a fast runner; in fact, her high school coach thought Alice would be fast enough to try out for the short dashes in the Olympics. He trained and timed her daily and her tests were good. She followed suggestions and her speech was adequate, constantly improving and understandable as she went to school, full time, five days a week.

All went well until September 1976 when her parents called to say that Alice had regressed. We had her come in for a blood sample and found that her

copper level had fallen to 60 mcg percent and her zinc
had risen to 300 mcg percent (iron was normal). We
theorized that this low copper and high zinc might be a
new cause for deviant behavior. I called her parents
and suggested that Alice be given daily one capsule of
a popular vitamin and mineral supplement which contains 2 mgm of copper. They were unconvinced and
waited a week before beginning the preparation. After
two days on the copper Alice was somewhat better,
and after a week she was once again training for the
dashes, hopefully for the future Olympics. Her copper
two months later was still in the sixties (62) but her
zinc was 120 mcg percent. She continues to improve.
We conclude that occasionally copper can go too low
and zinc too high on continued zinc diet supplementation.

Is Zinc a Good Tranquilizer in High Dosage? No!

The lad in Iran who ate his rocket fuel (10 grams of
metallic zinc) slept for five days and then recovered
without any lasting ill effects. Ordinarily we have not
used doses higher than 30 mgm of zinc as the gluconate three times per day. However, the parents of
Cindy, an eighteen-year-old girl, found on their own
that 1,000 to 5,000 mgm of zinc per day was calming,
so this dose of 20 to 100 tablets of 50 mgm zinc a day
was continued for several months. Cindy had been in a
psychiatric hospital for three months in 1974 without
benefit. She was found to be pyroluric in October 1975
and responded to zinc and B-6. However, while away
at college in early 1977, she stopped taking the zinc and
B-6 and became paranoid and delusional. Because of
the lack of results from her previous hospitalization,
her parents had attempted to treat her at home.

When seen on 10 June 1977 after two to three
months of taking 1,000 to 5,000 mgm zinc a day,
Cindy's serum zinc was 1,160 mcg percent (double-
checked) and her serum copper was 11 mcg percent
(rechecked four times). She had no detectable copper

protein (ceruloplasm) in her blood. Other pertinent data were blood white cells 3.9 thousand/cu mm with polys 18 percent and lymphocytes 76 percent. Her blood pressure was 100/60, pulse 120 and liver 1 cm below the costal margin. Her hemoglobin was 6.2 and red blood cell count 1.83 million/cu mm (normal 4.5), MCV (mean corpustular volume) 132 (normal 79 to 97). Cholesterol was 107 (normal 160), total serum protein 5.5 percent (normal 7.0), alk phos. 187 (normal below 110) and iron 55 mcg percent (normal 120). Her original histamine was a normal 57.4 nanog./ml, but with zinc intoxication the levels were 13.5 and, later, 0.0 nanog./ml. Spermidine was elevated by the zinc intoxication from 0.88 to 1.14, while spermine was initially reduced similar to the blood histamine. At the height of the zinc intoxication, the urine was normal, but two weeks later a specimen showed 1+ protein in the urine. She has slowly recovered; five weeks after the severe poisoning, her zinc is still 330 mcg percent, her copper only 17 mcg percent, with only a trace of the copper protein, ceruloplasm. The blood picture is now normal, although iron therapy was needed to improve her anemia. Her mental state remains good compared to her total psychosis before zinc and B-6 treatments.

Cindy's recovery from zinc poisoning was uneventful after the zinc intake was reduced to a reasonable amount. Her case demonstrates that zinc antagonizes body copper more than iron; that zinc lowers cholesterol; that polymorphonuclear white cells and red cells decrease, probably as a result of decreased formation. The original description of the body's need for copper was in the prevention of anemia, so we can understand the decrease in red cell count to 1.8 (normal 4.5), and the hemoglobin to 6.2 grams (normal 14 grams). As we go to press, we now know that her serum copper protein has returned to normal.

In retrospect, we might have anticipated that some parents might think that if some zinc were good a lot more would be better. We are fortunate to have these data on the effect of a large continued dose of zinc, but better data might have been collected under controlled conditions with more frequent monitoring of the trace metals and body chemistry. At present, we do not exceed 60 mgm of zinc (as the gluconate) four times per day in any of our patients. This dose is used only in those patients with high levels of serum copper and whose zinc, copper and iron is monitored at each visit. This report on zinc poisoning must be carefully weighed against zinc's benefits and against the alternate and ineffective therapy available for pyroluric patients now labeled schizophrenic.

"Zinc Deficiency Presenting as Schizophrenia"

This is the title of an article published by Drs. Staton, Donald and Green of the Psychiatric Institute of Columbia in Columbia, South Carolina in *Current Psychiatric Digest*. They point out the need to study zinc and copper relationships in psychotic patients.

Their zinc-deficient psychiatric patient was an eighteen-year-old male, A.G., a music major at a California college. Under emotional stress at college, the patient became agitated, and when admitted to a medical center he was found to be disoriented as to time and place and bothered by constant visual and auditory hallucinations. He did not respond to Prolixin 180 mgm per day or Haldol 100 mgm per day. He was returned to South Carolina and was committed for further study and treatment. The only laboratory abnormality was elevation of the liver enzymes SGOT, SGPT and LDH which rise with B-6 deficiency. The brain waves showed amorphous slow activity in all leads—again a sign of B-6 deficiency. Prolixin, Reserpine and Mellaril were administered without success. He had episodes of elevated blood pressure (150/120)—a sign of copper excess. He was delusional, hallucinating and self-destructive, and when questioned he slowly repeated the words of the examining doctor. A series of fifteen electroconvulsive treatments resulted in temporary improvement, but within ten days after ECT the patient was back to the original psychotic baseline and attempted to jump through a window.

Zinc Found to Be Low and Copper High

When all else failed, trace metal levels were run on the blood serum. The zinc was 65 mcg percent (normal 100 to 120) and copper was 185 (normal 100 mcg percent for males). In the words of the authors, "Because all other treatment had proven ineffective it was decided to treat the patient as if he were pyroluric and attempt to replace the zinc and pyridoxine."

On 160 mgm of zinc sulfate per day and 1 gram of B-6 twice a day, the patient became quiet in two days and more alert, and was able to leave his locked room and join the other patients in the ward. His muscle rigidity and tremor lessened in two days. Progress was steady, and within one month the patient was normal as to affect, plans for the future and knowledge of the world about him. His tested degree of insanity (Inpatient Behavior Scale) went from a high of 71 to a normal of 10 at discharge. Follow-up at three months showed continued improvement. Follow-up at one year found him back at college and doing well; his zinc level was still low (75 mcg percent) but his copper level was normal at 90 mcg percent. The patient cooperates fully and continues to take his daily dose of zinc and B-6.

The doctors conclude that they "believe that there exists a group of patients who have a zinc deficiency which, complicated by emotional stress, may present a schizophrenic picture. Because of the success and safety of the treatment it would seem worthwhile to attempt to identify and treat such patients." I can only say, "AMEN!"

If we compare the hazards of possible zinc toxicity when administered by overzealous parents with what eighteen-year-old A.G. went through before zinc was tried, there is a strong case for giving zinc and B-6 to *all* psychotic patients, whether they need it or not. Zinc and B-6 in moderate dosage can do no harm, whereas electroshock and jumping out of windows are definitely hazardous.

Sex and Zinc Update 1978

"If your libido lags check your zinc level"—so read the headline in a recent newspaper. But it is really not as simple as the oil dipstick on your auto engine. Zinc levels are not routinely measured by most hospital laboratories, and zinc varies with vitamin B-6 nutrition. Hence, the B-6 deficient patient may have a high serum zinc level because the zinc cannot be used without B-6. Zinc will do many things to lubricate the sexual machinery, such as: (1) increase penis and testes size in young growing males; (2) increase sperm motility; (3) decrease prostatitis and normalize secretion; (4) replace the zinc loss occasioned by excessive prostate secretion as in sexual foreplay and replace the zinc lost in the ejaculate; (5) help to prevent impotency. However the effect of zinc on the sexual drive or libido remains to be discovered. Zinc may contribute to the glint in the eye of the more aggressive mate since the retina and the prostate are both exceedingly high in zinc content. In the brain the pineal gland which regulates seasonal sex activity (rutting cycle) and the hippocampus which regulates emotions lead all other brain structures in zinc content. With all this knowledge we still cannot say that anyone's sex life would be better with excess zinc; we can only say that zinc is needed for normal sex activity, normal reproduction and the perfection of babies in all species. Let us then go to a practical update of what we really know.

Sperm Motility

Zinc is needed for the formation of active sperm and The prostate and prostatic secretions, and probably the normal ova in all mammalian species including man. vaginal secretions as well, are high in zinc content. In the final formation of active sperm, zinc is firmly bound within the keratin of the tail of the sperm. This keratin is similar to the horny layer or keratin layer of the skin which also contains and needs zinc for perfect formation. The zinc in both the skin and the sperm tail is firmly attached chemically to reduced sulfur in the form of sulfhydril groups. This keratin in the sperm accounts somehow for active motility. In a study of infertility, Drs. Stankovic and Mikac-Devic of Zagreb, Yugoslavia, found zinc levels of 20 mg percent in normal active semen, 14 mg percent in semen with decreased motility and 8 mg percent in semen without active sperm. All of the patient's *hair zinc* were within normal limits. The zinc-containing enzyme, acid phosphatase, showed similar decreases compared to the zinc levels as did also the level of cholesterol in the semen. In patients at the Brain Bio Center, we have been successful in increasing the fertility of childless couples by our nutrient program which includes zinc supplements. Cadmium as a pollutant or industrial poison decreases zinc levels in the testes and may be a factor in infertility.

Important Biochemicals in Semen

The trace metal content of human semen is of interest because of the prominence of zinc and sulfur. Calcium is 25 mg percent, zinc 20 mg percent, magnesium 14 mg percent, and copper only 0.05 mg percent, while sulfur is 3 percent of the ash. Potassium is only 89 mg percent while sodium is 281 mg percent, so semen tastes salty as the liberated generation has discovered. One patient asked whether she could swallow the semen, and the prompt reply was "of course, its very nutritious." These liberated days we have wives who claim that seminal nutrition is a good source of zinc; perhaps this opens a new market for the more voluminous boar semen. The odor of semen is due to amines such as spermine and spermidine. These chemicals come from the testes and are greatly diminished by vasectomy. The zinc content comes mainly from the prostate and is not diminished by vasectomy. The known vitamins in semen are inositol (54 mgm percent), vitamin C (13 mgm percent) and B-12 (300 to 600 nanogm percent). Important nutrients are citric acid (375 mgm percent), fructose (224 mgm percent), phosphorylcholine (315 mgm percent), cholesterol (80 mgm percent) and glutathione (30 mgm percent). We conclude that a high copper-low zinc diet might produce infertility, that inositol might be needed and that choline or its precursor deanol might help in some instances of male infertility.

Hypogonadism

The first description of zinc deficiency in man by Prasad listed small penis and scrotum as one of the cardinal signs of zinc deficiency in adolescents. This hypogonadism may not altogether distress the mother who dreads what her hyperactive son may do when he reaches sexual maturity, but the small penis-scrotum and lack of pubic hair creates psychological problems for the adolescent boy. At school after sports activities, boys shower together and the boy with small penis is apt to be ridiculed by those who are better equipped. This leads to lasting doubts as to whether or not the penis is big enough to satisfy a female.

Fortunately, the effects of zinc deficiency on the male gonads are completely reversible as has been shown in man, the sheep, and the rat. As early as 1969, Drs. E. J. Underwood and M. Somers of Australia found that young rams who were severely zinc-deficient would not mount females, nor could they collect active sperm from the animals. The animals had no libido but then they also had eczema of the face and scrotum, and lost their horns and wool as a result of the severe zinc deficiency. All of these signs of zinc deficiency disappeared when zinc was added to the diet. After twenty weeks on zinc, the sperm count of the zinc-repleted rams equaled that of the control rams. Dr. Lucille Hurley and her group in California have made similar observations on rats on a zinc-deficient diet. Symptoms of skin ulcers began in one week and were severe in two weeks. The deficient diet was fed for twenty-eight days and then the animals were repleted with a zinc-sufficient diet. Partial reversal occurred in six days and complete reversal in fifteen days. These studies should reassure the adolescent who has hypogonadism and even breast swelling (gynecomastia), that help is on the way with dietary zinc and adequate B-6 to produce dream recall.

Can Masturbation Cause Zinc Deficiency?

Dr. John C. Boursnell of Cambridge, England works with male pigs (boars) and writes that the single ejaculate of the boar may contain as much as 12 mgm of zinc! The boar weighs up to 100 kgm, or about twice as much as an adolescent youth. The 12 mgm of zinc in the single ejaculate of the boar almost equals the amount of zinc that each individual should get each day in the so-called well-rounded diet (which doesn't exist!). So what do we know about zinc loss from sex or masturbation in man?

First, we hasten to add that the single ejaculate of the boar may equal a half pint of fluid or 300 ml; the human ejaculate measures 4.5 ml. Man loses more fluid in petting or foreplay prior to ejaculation; this secretion is prostatic fluid which is high in zinc content. The content of zinc in good human semen is 20 mgm percent or 20 mgm per 100 ml. If the ejaculate were 5 ml, the loss of zinc in each ejaculate might total as much as 1 mgm, which is less startling than that of the boar. With marathon necking and petting, the loss of zinc again might equal 1 mgm since normal prostate fluid has 0.5 mgm per ml or 50 mgm percent, according to Drs. William R. Fair and W. Heston of the Washington School of Medicine in St. Louis. With these figures in mind, the zinc loss would be greatest in any sex activity with extended foreplay. We hate to say it but in a zinc-deficient adolescent, sexual excitement and excessive masturbation might precipitate insanity. I do recall that puritanical official from the YMCA who talked to the segregated high school boys and stated that the grey stuff from the penis was equal to the loss of the same amount of grey matter from the brain each time we masturbated.

Zinc and Prostatitis

Drs. Fair and Heston found that in prostatitis the level of zinc was one-tenth the level in normal glands and that the prostatitis responded slowly to an extra dietary supplement of zinc as the gluconate salt. S. Colleen, et al. found that the zinc level of semen was significantly lower in gonnococcal bacterial infections (six patients). Chronic infection or stress of any kind is known to lower the blood serum zinc level. Chronic prostatitis in middle-aged men is a debilitating disorder which may continue for months and years during which time antibiotics are continually tried in hopes of effecting a cure. Certainly, zinc gluconate should be used as a dietary supplement as an aid to rid the body of this nagging infection.

Benign Prostatic Hypertrophy

As man ages, the prostate gets bigger, a phenomenon that also occurs in male dogs and perhaps in other species. The 4 plus enlargement of the prostate results in urinary obstruction, and with the retention of urine, bladder infections may occur. Some men may need an operation before the age of sixty, yet I have one patient, in good nutrition, who at ninety-four has not had a prostate operation. He now takes zinc gluconate 30 mgm A.M. and P.M. and 0.3 mgm of conjugated estrogens each day. The female sex hormone is frequently helpful in reducing the size of the enlarged prostate. Zinc, when balanced with other trace elements and vitamins, is probably helpful in preventing cancer of the prostate and breast.

References

Boursnell, J. C. Personal communication. Agricultural Research Council, Cambridge, England, 1972.

Byar, D. P.; Anderson, J. E. and Mostofi, F. K. The distribution of zinc in the prostate and other organs in control, castrated, and hypophysectomized rats. *Investigative Urology* 7(1):57–65, 1969.

Calvin, H. I. and Bleau, G. Zinc-thiol complexes in keratin-like structures of rat spermatozoa. *Experimental Cell Research* 86:280–284, 1974.

Calvin, H. I., Hwang, F. H. and Herma Wohlrab, H. Localization of zinc in a dense fiber-connecting piece fraction of rat sperm tails analogous chemically to hair keratin. *Biology of Reproduction* 13:228–239, 1975.

Colleen, S.; Mardh, P. A. and Schytz, A. Magnesium and zinc in seminal fluid of healthy males and patients with non-acute prostatitis with and without gonorrhoea. *Scandinavian Journal of Urology & Nephrology* 9:192–197, 1975.

Diamond, I.; Swenerton, H. and Hurley, L. S. Testicular and esophageal lesions in zinc-deficient rats and their reversibility. *Journal of Nutrition* 101:77–84, 1971.

Eliasson, R.; Johnsen, O. and Lindholmer, C. Effect of zinc on human sperm respiration. *Life Sciences* 10(1):1317–1320, 1971.

Eliasson, R. and Lindholmer, C. Zinc in human seminal plasma. Reproductive Physiology Unit, Karolinska Institute, Stockholm, Sweden, 1971.

Fair, W. R. Prostate inflammation linked to zinc shortage. *Prevention* 113:June 1977.

Heston, W. Prostate inflammation linked to zinc shortage. *Prevention* 113:June 1977.

Jameson, S. Variations in maternal serum zinc during pregnancy and correlation to congenital malformations, dysmaturity, and abnormal parturition, effects of zinc deficiency in human reproduction. *Linkoping University Medical Dissertations* 37:1976.

Janick, J.; Zeitz, L. and Whitemore, W. Seminal fluid and spermatozoon zinc levels and their relationship to human spermatozoon motility. *Fertility and Sterility* 22(9): 573–589, 1971.

Kesseru, E. and Leon, F. Effect of different solid metals and metallic pairs on human sperm motility. *International Journal of Fertility* 19:81–84, 1974.

Mann, T. *The biochemistry of semen and of the male reproductive tract*. New York: John Wiley & Sons, 1974.

Stankovic, H. and Mikac-Devic, D. Zinc and copper in human semen. *Clinica Chimica Acta* 70:123–126, 1976.

Underwood, E. J. and Somers, M. Studies of zinc nutrition in sheep. I. The relation of zinc to growth, testicular development, and spermatogenesis in young rams. *Australian Journal of Agricultural Research* 20:889–897, 1969.

Webb, M.; Creed, H. and Atkinson, S. Influence of zinc on protein synthesis by polyribosomes from the dog prostate and the dorsolateral lobes of the rat prostate. *Biochimica et Biophysica Acta* 324:143–155, 1973.

What Can Zinc Plus Pyridoxine Do for You?

Salt and pepper has been used to season food through the ages, but with all the junk foods and empty calories that are being consumed today we suggest that they be seasoned with zinc and pyridoxine (B-6). In contrast to whole grain bread, the white flour roll contains little zinc, and the soft drink, compared to milk, contains no B-6. Both zinc and B-6 are needed to cope with the stress of modern life. If you do not have zinc and B-6 in adequate amounts, at an early age you will probably develop acne, headaches, stomach aches, impotency, missed menstrual periods, itching in sunlight, inability to suntan, stretch marks, white spotted finger nails, no dream recall, anemia, painful knees, fruity breath, tremors, spasms, elevated blood pressure, amnesia—and perhaps get spaced out—a psychosis!

As you finger your worry beads and live miserably through one or more of these aggravating ailments, you may still die young from stroke, heart attack or cancer. With such prospects for the future, who would want to live on jiffy foods when nature provides a better life on natural foods with zinc and B-6? Let us now review some of the data that have been accumulated on zinc and B-6. We found that the mauve factor (krypto-pyrrole, KP) takes zinc and B-6 into the urine, so the body is constantly robbed and even more so with stress of any kind. Since about 10 to 15 percent of all people excrete the mauve factor, their need for zinc and B-6 may far exceed their need for salt and pepper.

The National Research Council has approved the addition of small amounts of zinc and B-6 to white flour, but as slowly as a glacier moves, the bureaucracy will take years to implement the suggestion—and even then cosmetic and cost factors may further stall the endeavor. The proposed level of enrichment for cereal-grain products is 2.2 mcg percent for zinc and 0.44 mcg percent for pyridoxine. These levels are found in most natural whole grain foods.

Man needs to absorb 15 mgm of zinc every day, but our best diets give only 8 to 11 mgm; hospital diets may provide even lower amounts. Man needs 2 mgm of B-6 per day (1 quart of milk), but in times of stress the need for B-6 soars so that some patients who excrete the mauve factor in their urine may need 500 mgm of B-6 A.M. and P.M. Normal dream recall depends on an adequate amount of B-6 in the brain. With too much B-6 the individual may be awakened with a vivid dream every two hours during the night. This is not harmful in itself; it is simply nature's way of telling us to take slightly less B-6. Some adults think that only children dream, but this is not so; almost all adults will remember their dreams if they are given enough B-6. Some may consider dreams trivial and unimportant, but we say dream recall is normal and is a good test of whether or not your recent memory is working.

Let us consider a few of the diseases that are cured by zinc and B-6. Please note that I seldom use the word cure except for cheese and tobacco. When a vitamin or trace element deficiency is corrected, we can then logically use the word *cure*.

Acne

When parakeratosis, the skin disorder of pigs, was proven in 1955 to be a zinc deficiency, a farmer in West Virginia suggested to the family doctor that zinc might also relieve his son's aggravated acne. The farmer was right and the acne cleared. Further support for zinc in skin conditions came with a lethal rare skin disease which occurs in infants at weaning, acrodermatitis enteropathica (AE). These AE infants develop infections around every body orifice when shifted from mother's milk to milk formula. All formulas are low in zinc content and some, when diluted with tap water, may be high in copper. With the knowledge that acne could be the result of zinc deficiency at puberty, many doctors are using zinc preparations effectively for acne. A letter to the editor of the *Australian Medical Journal* in 1976 was entitled *Is Acne Vulgaris Zinc Deficiency?* The final word arrived from Sweden via the AMA, *Archives for Dermatology* (January 1977), in which Dr. Gerd Michaelsson of Uppsala University compared vitamin A alone, zinc alone, both zinc and vitamin A and a dummy capsule in four groups of acne patients. The acne decreased only in the two zinc-treated groups where the acne score went from 85 down to 15 pimples per group; the vitamin A (in butter-eating Swedes) gave no added improvement. This finding confirms what many family physicians have found with simple zinc supplementation of the diet. During the stressful years of puberty, zinc is needed for ovarian function, growth, the prostate, seminal vesicles, testes and in sperm production. The ejaculate of the boar contains 12 mgm of zinc and that of man 15 mcg percent. Small wonder, then, that simple masturbation may sometimes aggravate zinc deficiency.

Rheumatoid Arthritis Responds Slowly to Zinc

The Brain Bio Center has used zinc and other nutrients in the treatment of rheumatoid arthritis since 1971 when a fifty-seven-year-old-male patient presented with a serum copper level of 144, zinc of 74 and iron of 56 mcg percent. With zinc therapy his copper level crested at 174 in two months, his zinc rose to a constant 94 and his iron has never again been so low. His latest copper levels are around 110 to 115 mcg percent. He has been able to continue his work as a cabinet maker.

Younger arthritic patients with high copper and low zinc levels have benefited even more rapidly. Professor Peter A. Simkin, a rheumatologist at the University of Washington Medical School in Seattle, noted the low zinc and low histidine levels in rheumatoid arthritic patients and decided to do something about it. He gave 220 mgm of zinc sulfate three times a day to twelve rheumatoid arthritic patients and dummy capsules to another twelve patients for twelve weeks. After that, all patients got zinc for another twelve-week period. With zinc, significant improvement occurred in walking, stiffness and inflammation of the joints, and in the patients' opinions most felt better. With this therapy the zinc-containing enzyme alkaline phosphatase rose from 79 to 96 units/liter. The patients' blood histidine fell from a low of 1.57 mcg percent to an ever greater low of 1.36 mcg percent (normal is 180 mcg percent). Obviously, in Dr. Simkin's next trial he will use both the amino acid l-histidine and the micro nutrient zinc. As has been proven in past studies, no symptom of intoxication occurred in this study other than mild diarrhea. We hope that other internists will now use zinc and perhaps l-histidine in their rheumatoid arthritic patients. L-histidine chelates many divalent metals such as copper, zinc, iron and calcium. While we believe the mode of action of zinc is to drive copper and iron from the inflamed joints, this is only one group's theory since zinc also influences infection and immune reactions in the body.

Zinc and Infection

Patients who are zinc-deficient have body swelling which even extends to the face to involve the hollow sinuses and tubes. As a result of swollen air passages the patients have a constant nasal twang which goes away when zinc and B-6 are given. Even nasal polyps are resorbed in some patients with zinc and B-6.

In children, the swollen face of zinc deficiency also extends to the auditory tubes that drain the inner ear which, when open, allow the air pressure to equalize and fluids to drain. When swollen shut, the middle ear can become infected, resulting in earache and pus behind the ear drum. Children with recurrent middle ear infections do not have these infections when they get adequate amounts of zinc and vitamin B-6. In this instance, the control of infection is partly mechanical because of relief of the swollen tissues, but zinc has other actions which enhance immunity and may be directly bacteriocidal.

Bacteriocidal Effect of Zinc

Professor Galask and his colleagues at the University of Iowa Medical School, curious as to why the bag of waters in pregnant women seldom becomes infected, have found that zinc works closely with a simple polypeptide which contains, for its amino acids, one lysine, one glycine and three glutamic acid molecules. This bacterial inhibitor requires zinc (about 250 mcg percent) and a low level of phosphate. High levels of phosphate support *E. Coli* growth, while higher levels of zinc are even more bacteriocidal in the presence of the polypeptide. We do not yet know if this polypeptide occurs elsewhere in the body, but the chances are that it does.

We have found that zinc-deficient pyroluric patients are very prone to many types of infection, including viruses such as herpes simplex. Characteristically, their differential white blood cell count shows an immature distribution, namely high lymphocytes and low poly or segmented cells. Eosinophils may be as high as 25 percent in pyroluria. With zinc and B-6, the polys go to the usual 70 percent and the eosinophilia goes down to 1 percent or less. Dr. A. Prasad and his co-workers in

Detroit have found a similar blood cell picture with zinc deficiency.

Zinc and B-6 Are Needed to Fight Infection

At the Brain Bio Center we have found that the hyperactive or autistic child invariably has high copper and low zinc levels. Other heavy metals may be as great a stimulant to the brain as is copper. Some researchers have discovered lead levels to be moderately high, as have we, but the main source of stimulation seems to be any combination of metals such as copper, lead, mercury and perhaps silver.

Dr. Moynihan of London has noted the striking similarity of the AE baby to the autistic child. Zinc is important in the retina and lack of zinc makes direct vision painful; thus the child uses his peripheral vision to greet visitors. The first sign of the effectiveness of zinc in both AE and autism is the sunrise of a great direct smile from the usually diffident youngster. Drs. Stubbs and Crawford of Portland, Oregon, have found depressed lymphocyte responsiveness in the autistic child. When the cells in culture are challenged with a hemagglutinin (PHA), the response is significantly less than that of the age-matched controls, which indicates an inadequate lymphocyte immune response.

Dr. M. Chvapil and his colleagues from Arizona have discovered that lymphocytes from animals on a high zinc diet are most susceptible to PHA. This indicates the biochemical need for zinc in the autistic child. Chvapil has reported that the phagocytes of the body with high zinc content are less active. Dr. Phillips of San Antonio, Texas, has noted that zinc transferrin is normally bound to lymphocytes and that this zinc transport system may be a vital beginning in immune reactions.

Dr. Robert S. Pecarek of the Trace Metal Laboratory, following the lead that the thymus is always small in zinc-deficient animals, has found that T-cell immunity is impaired. The fact that lymphocytes from the thymus gland have most to do with defense against viruses might explain the severity and long duration of infectious mononucleosis in some individuals. The "kissing disease" is ordinarily a self-limited infection but in patients whose resistance is low hepatitis and even encephalitis can result.

Several years ago, we listed Reye's Syndrome as a possible complication of flu in copper-excess, zinc-deficient patients. The treatment for Reye's Syndrome is total blood exchange. Red blood cells are high in zinc which may be the curative agent.

Drs. Airgad and Bernheimer of New York City have found that zinc prevents the hemolysis produced by bacterial toxins, and Dr. J. E. Repine and his co-workers of Minnesota have described a patient with repeated infections who had a very low level of alkaline phosphatase in the white blood cells. Alkaline phosphatase is one of the more than twenty enzymes in the human body that require zinc for normal function.

TABLE 1.4

Acrodermatitis enteropathica—symptoms
Human Zinc Deficiency

Erythematous and pustular dermatitis on neck, face, trunk, buttocks, legs and around all body orifices

Alopecia—complete loss of hair

Diarrhea

Retardation of growth and sexual development

Amenorrhea or impotency

Lactose intolerance

Finger and toenail changes and infections

Dental caries

Conjunctivitis and photophobia—indirect gaze

High blood pressure

Increased susceptibility to infection

Impaired development of immune system

Gynecomastia—breast growth in males

Lassitude and muscle weakness

Behavior changes—disperceptions and confusion

This rare disease exemplifies many of the symptoms of zinc deficiency in man. The disease responds dramatically to extra dietary zinc.

TABLE 1.5

Some food sources of vitamin B-6

Brewer's yeast	2.50 mgm%
Sunflower seeds	1.25 mgm%
Wheat germ	1.15 mgm%
Liver	0.84 mgm%
Fresh meat	0.55 mgm%
Soybeans	0.81 mgm%
Salmon	0.70 mgm%
Lentils	0.60 mgm%
Brown rice	0.55 mgm%
Chickpeas	0.54 mgm%
Chicken	0.32 mgm%
Green vegetables	0.20 mgm%
Milk	2.00 mgm% per quart
Eggs	0.11 mgm%

In general, good food sources of B-6 are hard to find in nature. Note, however, that brewer's yeast has 2.5 mgm per 100 grams—a whole day's supply, if one can tolerate 3 ounces (100 gms) of brewer's yeast. Note that sunflower seeds and wheat germ can substitute for brewer's yeast. The mauve factor pyroluric patient requires 50 to 500 mgm size tablets of B-6 each day. This daily dose is enough to produce dream recall each night.

Summary

We have given several cogent reasons why you should now substitute zinc and B-6 and natural foods for the salt and pepper of jiffy food existence. Obviously, other vitamins and micro nutrients may be needed, but these are more easily available from natural whole grain foods. Try zinc and B-6 for starters. You may find your eyes opened wider, your ears unplugged and your dreams realized with just one week of zinc and B-6 supplementation of your diet.

References

Avigad, L. S. and Bernheimer, A. W. Inhibition by zinc hemolysis induced by bacterial and other cytolytic agents. *Infection and Immunity* 13(5):1378–1381, 1976.

Gartside, J. M. and Allen, B. R. Treatment of acrodermatitis enteropathica with zinc sulphate. *Br. Med. J.* 3:521–522, 1975.

Michaelsson, G. Effects of oral zinc and vitamin A in acne. *JAMA Archives for Dermatology* 113:3–36, 1977.

Moynihan, E. J. Zinc deficiency and disturbances of mood and visual behavior. *The Lancet* 1/10:91, 1976.

Pecarek, R. S.; Powanda, M. C. and Hoagland, A. M. Effect of zinc deficiency on the immune response of the rat. *Fed. Proc.* 35:360, 1976.

Pfeiffer, C. C. *Mental and elemental nutrients.* New Canaan, Connecticut: Keats Publishing, 1975.

Phillips, J. C. Specific binding of zinc transferrin to human lymphocytes. *Biochemical and Biophysical Research Communications* 72(2):634–639, 1976.

Prasad, A. S.; Abbasi, A.; Oberleas, D.; Rabbani, P.; Fernandez-Madrid, F. and Ryan, J. Experimental production of zinc deficiency in man. *Fed. Proc.* 35;658, 1976.

Repine, J. E., et al. Primary leukocyte alkaline phosphatase deficiency in adult with repeated infections. *Br. J. Haematol.* 34:87–95, 1976.

Schlievert, P.; Johnson, W. and Galask, R. Bacterial growth inhibition by amniotic fluid. *Am. J. Obstet. Gynecol.* 127:603, 1977.

Simkin, P. A. Oral zinc sulphate in rheumatoid arthritis. *The Lancet* 9/11:539–542, 1976.

Stankova, L.; Drach, G. W.; Hicks, T.; Zukoski, C. F. and Chvapil, M. Regulation of some functions of granulocytes by zinc of the prostatic fluid and prostate tissue. *J. of Lab. and Clin. Med.* 88(4):640–648, 1976.

Stubbs, E. G.; Crawford, M. G.; Burger, D. R. and Vandonbark, A. A. Depressed lymphocytes responsiveness in autistic children. *Journal of Autism and Childhood Schizophrenia* 7(1):49–55, 1977.

CHAPTER 2

Iron

IRON is essential to human body chemistry, since it combines with protein to make hemoglobin, the coloring matter of red blood cells. The body makes efficient use of iron stores by "recycling," but when blood is lost through menstruation or hemorrhage, iron is also lost and must be replaced by adequate dietary intake. If this deficiency is not adjusted, an anemia may result.

The similarity between iron-deficiency anemia and other anemias, particularly pyridoxal-deficiency anemia, presents the possibility of an iron accumulation overload when iron is given in abundance. Doctors who fear incipient iron-deficiency anemia or who misdiagnose another deficiency may prescribe iron supplements for their patients. Current advertising warns consumers of the danger of iron deficiency, with the result that self-medication with products like Geritol, Hadacol, Ironized Yeast and One-a-day Vitamins Plus Iron is not uncommon. This adds up to too much "TV iron" for some people.

Iron deficiency is more likely to occur in women than in men, and in teen-agers whose rapid growth may require additional iron. In pregnancy and cases of overt blood loss, the risk of deficiency is enough to merit supplements. Iron overload is most likely to occur in older men, as the excess iron accumulates gradually over the years. The individual who has fortified himself with daily doses of "TV iron" for the last thirty years is a likely candidate for iron overload. As with copper, excess iron can have pernicious consequences. Among these are hemachromatosis or siderosis (an iron-excess disease), damage to the liver and pancreas, arthritis and heart damage.

Bread and cereals are usually fortified with iron, but there are much better choices of nutrients to add. Pyridoxine (B-6) and zinc are two such nutrients. A deficiency of these can cause blood disorders which mimic iron deficiency. Based only on hemoglobin levels, some claim that iron deficiency is our most critical nutritional problem. We believe that deficiency in B-6 and zinc is more critical.

Excess tissue iron is more insidious than iron deficiency. It develops gradually over the years, potentially developing into hemosiderosis or hemochromatosis. In those already suffering from hemochromatosis, thalassemia or sickle cell disease, the extra iron can be fatal. Because iron-deficiency anemia may sometimes be confused with other anemias, the best way to diagnose an iron deficiency is by measuring the serum iron level, *not* the hemoglobin. The propensity to equate "iron deficiency" with "anemia" is responsible for much of the present controversy.

Types of Anemia

An anemia is any one of many disorders which involve a reduction in the concentration of hemoglobin (number of red blood cells per unit volume of blood). It results in a decreased ability of the blood to carry oxygen. Symptoms include weakness, pallor, loss of appetite and the wide array of symptoms which may occur with any disease underlying anemia.

The breakdown of hemoglobin takes place constantly, and iron from this is added to the absorption iron and to the iron released from body reserves which is needed to maintain homeostasis. Iron is withdrawn from the plasma into the bone marrow and synthesized into new hemoglobin with the aid of copper as a catalyst. The life cycle of a red blood cell is about 120 days.

Iron deficiency is often without symptoms other than those associated with anemia of any cause. The establishment of a diagnosis involves measurement of the plasma iron concentration and the iron-binding capacity of the carrier protein, transferrin. It must also be demonstrated that iron stores have been completely depleted. The patient's history must also be scrutinized and a demonstrable blood loss should be sought. This may occur in regular blood donors and those with a history of gastrointestinal bleeding (sometimes due to salicylates such as aspirin, and other drugs). Growing children and women during the reproductive years are most susceptible to blood-loss anemia.

Iron-deficiency anemia rarely constitutes a life-threatening predicament. Patients can walk with only 20 percent of their normal hemoglobin. The first thing which is treated is the cause of the blood loss. Then body iron is replenished, usually by an oral preparation. If the hemoglobin level does not steadily rise (at least 2 gm per 100 ml of blood for every three weeks of therapy), it is possible that the anemia is not caused by iron deficiency.

Pyridoxine-deficiency (or pyridoxal-responsive) anemia may be mistaken for iron-deficiency anemia. Here, however, the serum iron level is often elevated and bone marrow hemosiderin increased. Then, in addition to pernicious anemia (for which there is no cure but which is controlled by periodic doses of folic acid and B-12), there are the significant anemias of blood loss, of protein deficiency, of kidney failure and of liver failure, which must be differentiated from iron deficiency.

Excess Iron

When an excessive amount of iron is ingested frequently over long periods, several pathological conditions of far greater life-threatening potential than those of iron deficiency can arise. An example is the hemosiderosis found in the Northern Veld Bantu tribe of

South Africa. These tribesmen used iron pots for preparation of beer and sour porridge. Since these foods are acidic, the iron can leach out into them. Adult Bantu males, who drank large quantities of this beer, had a high incidence of hemosiderosis and scurvy. The scurvy was due to the irreversible oxidation of ascorbic acid by the tissue iron deposits. These men were also susceptible to liver injury and may have shown evidence of liver scarring (cirrhosis).

Hemosiderosis is a disease of the iron metabolism characterized by deposits of iron in the liver. Typical symptoms of cirrhosis may evolve from this. The transferrin (iron-carrying transport protein) becomes saturated with iron and is no longer able to bind all of the absorbed iron. Excess iron may end up in the lungs, pancreas and heart, as well as the liver. The daily iron intake among Bantu men ranges from 30 mg to 100 mg, so it comes as no surprise that the disease may occur after any prolonged therapy with unneeded iron.

Iron-storage disease may result from a serum iron level permanently elevated by prolonged medicinal iron in the form of oral preparations or injections. Other sources include extensive blood transfusion, presence of other disease, hemolytic anemia, aplastic anemia and early acute hepatitis. All are characterized by high iron levels. A strict vegetarian regime may also produce iron overloading.

The iron-overloading diseases are basically an inability of the digestive tract to screen out unneeded iron. They appear mostly in men over the age of forty, and symptoms include headache, shortness of breath, increasing fatigue, dizziness and loss of weight. The iron becomes deposited in the tissues, and in time the iron deposits give the skin a grey hue. While heredity may contribute to disposition of some toward the disease, a high intake of iron appears to be the main cause. Persons who drink large quantities of iron-containing red wine, and persons who are addicted to certain iron tonics have a proclivity toward acquisition of the disease.

One organ in which iron deposits may accumulate is

the heart. Cardiac iron deposits which are easily visible at autopsy occur in patients with idiopathic hemochromatosis. Another place the iron ends up is the synovial membrane of the rheumatoid joints. Studies have shown a disturbance in iron metabolism among arthritic patients, and although no cause-effect relationship has been shown, it is possible that the synovial membranes are acting as storage depots for excess iron. Dr. K. D. Muirden has hypothesized that regional lymph nodes in rheumatoid arthritis are areas of iron storage.

Iron overload often goes unnoticed due to the fervor associated with the elimination of iron deficiency. Pyridoxine- and zinc-deficiency syndromes may be responsible for the anemia or other condition, and in these cases a daily dose of iron is not the nicest thing you can do for yourself.

Ninety percent of the dietary iron intake remains unabsorbed, never even entering the blood. There is a small daily excretion in the urine and feces, from menstruation, in perspiration and in exfoliation of the skin which requires replacement from dietary sources. Extra dietary iron is required when blood volume expands (as with rapid growth or development of the fetus) or when blood loss occurs.

Sources of Iron

Lean meats, deep-green leaf vegetables, whole-grain cereals or breads, liver, other organ meats, dried fruits, legumes, shell-fish and molasses are rich in iron. Iron cookware is another source, although iron skillets are generally the only such items still in use since the advent of aluminum, copper and stainless steel. The daily requirement of iron is probably twice as great in women and adolescents than in men, but pregnancy is the only general condition for which iron supplementation is recommended. Again, the general population would benefit more from more B-6 and zinc supplementation than from more iron.

References

Arora, R.; Lynch, E. C.; Whitly, C. E.; Alfrey, E., Jr. and Clarence, P. The ubiquity and significance of human ferratin. *Texas Rep. Biol. Med.* 28:3, 189–196, 1970.

Brody, K. and Will, G. Iron absorption in rheumatoid arthritis. *Annals of the rheumatoid diseases* 28:5. September 1969.

Crosby, W. H. Intestinal response to the body's requirement for iron. *JAMA* 208:2, 347–351, 14 April 1969.

Goodman, L. S. and Gilman, A. *The pharmacological basis of therapeutics.* New York: Macmillan, 1955.

Muirden, K. D. The anemia of rheumatoid arthritis: the significance of iron deposits in the synovial membrane. *Aust. Ann. Med.* 2:97–104, 1970.

——Lymph node iron in rheumatoid arthritis. *Annals of Rheumatic Diseases* 29:1, January 1970.

Robinson, C. H. *Fundamentals of normal nutrition.* New York: Macmillan, 1973.

Siimes, M. A., Addiego, J. E., Jr. and Dallman, P. R. Ferratin in serum: diagnosis of iron deficiency and iron overload in infants and children. *Blood* 43:4, April 1974.

Iron Update 1978

In the good old days, if you were pale and fatigued grandma would first try sulfur and molasses (high in iron) and if this didn't work she might have tried a special remedy. At night she would stick some rusty nails into an apple and let the spiked apple sit overnight. The next day you would be ordered to eat the whole apple—naturally removing the nails first! Presumably, the apple solubilized the iron which was then better absorbed. Research has revealed that iron absorption in the human body is more complex than grandma would have guessed, but acids such as malic and ascorbic in the apple do promote absorption. For this reason, iron-deficiency anemia is variably responsive to iron supplements depending on what is eaten with the iron. In a study of 300 pregnant women, dosages of 100 to 200 mgs of ferrous sulfate resulted in the same rise in hemoglobin levels. Other nutritional factors affect iron absorption. Vitamin C supplements increase iron retention significantly, and eggs and orange juice in the morning are recognized as a nutritionally advantageous combination. Vitamin C in the orange juice chelates and reduces the iron of the egg yolk, facilitating its absorption. An unbalanced vegetarian diet or excess consumption of phosphate in the diet results in less iron absorbed. The toxic metals lead, cadmium or copper reduce iron absorption.

Iron Fortification

Iron-deficiency anemia is often cited as the world's number one nutritional problem. Iron fortification of salt and dehydrated potatoes has been recommended, and preliminary laboratory testing is underway. The difficulty in predicting the degree of iron absorption in various populations suggests that it is unreasonable to further fortify common household foods. Iron problems must be treated on a more individual basis, and the treatment of anemia must certainly be individualized.

Treatment of Excess Iron

Diseases of iron poisoning, overload or excess storage can result from dietary or genetic causes. Chelated minerals or agents such as 2,3 dihydroxybenzoic acid and deferoxamine mesylate successfully purge the body of toxic iron via the urine.

References

Chandra, R. K. Iron and immunocompetence. *Nutrition Reviews* 34:129–135, 1976.

Cooley's Anemia Therapy. *Medical Doctor:* 68, June 1977.

Grebe, G., et al. Effects of meals and ascorbic acid on the

absorption of a therapeutic dose of iron as ferrous and ferric salts. *Current Therapeutic Research* 17:382–397, 1975.

King, R. D., et al. Transferrin iron and dermatophytes I. *Journal of Laboratory and Clinical Medicine* 86:204–212, 1975.

Layrisse, M. Dietary iron absorption. *Nutrition* 1:141–148, 1975.

Lukens, J. N. Iron deficiency and infection. *Am J. Dis. Child* 129:160–162, 1975.

Peterson, C. M. Chelation studies with 2, 3, dihydroxybenzoic acid in patients with thalessemia major. *JAMA* 236:2691, 1976.

Physical acceptability and bioavailability of iron fortified food. *Nutrition Reviews* 34:298–300, 1976.

Sjosedt, J. E., et al. Oral iron prophylaxis during pregnancy: a comparative study on different dosage regimens. *Acta Obstetricia et Gynecologica Scandinavica* 60:3–9, 1977.

Skin Plants: denying them iron. *Science News*, 3 May 1975.

Underwood, E. J. *Trace elements in human and animal nutrition.* New York: Academic Press, 1977.

CHAPTER 3

Manganese

THE high copper level of many schizophrenics can be reduced by dietary intake of zinc and manganese. Manganese is similar to zinc in the way it increases urinary copper excretion; a combination of zinc and manganese is more effective than either alone. High-copper schizophrenics are improved by the zinc-manganese combination in Ziman drops or tablets.

Manganese is one of the essential trace metals, a necessary dietary constituent obtained from nuts, seeds, and whole-grain cereals. It is necessary for bone growth and development, reproduction, lipid metabolism and the moderation of nervous irritability. Manganese is also important in the building and breakdown cycles of protein and nucleic acid (the chief carrier of genetic information). As an activator of such enzymes as arginase (required for the formation of urea) and some peptidases (which cause the hydrolysis of proteins in the intestine), manganese may also contribute to a mother's love and instinctive maternal protection of her child. (Through certain enzymes, manganese affects the glandular secretions underlying maternal instinct.) Manganese is important in the formation of thyroxin, the principle of the thyroid gland.

Required Intake

Every day a healthy person excretes approximately 4 mg of manganese; this amount is then needed in the diet for replacement of the lost manganese. Adequate intake is required for the lipid and glucose metabolism and oxidative phosphorylation (among other intrinsic biochemical processes). On normal lipid metabolism manganese has a beneficial effect, particularly in cases of atherosclerosis.

Manganese Deficiency

Analysis of hair samples has indicated that manganese deficiency may be common among older males. Manganese deficiency may be a cause of atherosclerosis, although no studies have clearly demonstrated a true deficiency of this trace metal in man. Similarly, manganese deficiency is suspected in diabetes. A study by L. G. Kosenko in 1964 implicated manganese deficiency after an examination of 122 diabetics from fifteen to eighty-one years of age. Dr. Kosenko found that the manganese content of whole ashed blood was approximately half that of normal control subjects. In 1968 G. J. Everson and R. E. Shrader reported that manganese deficiency can impair the glucose metabolism so as to lower glucose tolerance (the ability to remove excess sugar from the blood). The deficiency may produce abnormalities in the pancreatic secretion of insulin, the agent which utilizes excess sugar. Thus, a diabetic condition may result.

The enzymes which manganese activates are also necessary for the utilization of vitamin C, choline and other B vitamins (biotin and thiamin). Without the ability to use choline or deanol properly, the body underproduces acetylcholine, a neurotransmitter in the brain. In a body deficient in acetylcholine and properly utilized B vitamins, various conditions may result, among them myasthenia gravis (grave loss of muscle strength). This condition may respond to manganese if doses are given at each meal, in addition to a high-protein diet, vitamin E and all the B vitamins. All these nutrients aid in the transmission of impulses between nerve and muscle.

Poisoning

Manganese overloading or poisoning has been reported only in industries where manganese-containing dust may be inhaled. In mining operations in Chile and in the dry battery industry, where workers are exposed to manganese oxide dust, cases of manganese poisoning have been recorded. Symptoms are similar to those of Parkinsonism and include tremor, muscular rigidity, irritability and impotency. Symptoms of chronic manganese poisoning in these industries may also resemble those of schizophrenia. A drug used in treating Parkinson's disease, 1-dopa (dihydroxyphenylalanine) has been found useful in treating manganese overload.

Metabolism

Manganese metabolism is somewhat similar to that of iron. Manganese is absorbed slowly from the small intestine, and the unneeded portion is excreted. The absorbed portion is transported through the blood by the protein transmanganin; the manganese quickly leaves the bloodstream and is stored mainly in the kidney. Some is excreted in the urine, most into the bile.

Manganese and Schizophrenia

Manganese chloride was first tested and found effective in treating schizophrenia by Dr. Reiter of Denmark. This finding was confirmed in 1929 by Dr. W. M. English, superintendent of a hospital in Brockville, Ontario. A later study by Hoskins, however, found manganese dioxide ineffective and since then, little attention has focused on the possibility of its therapeutic effects. The finding of high copper levels in the schizophrenias has also been ignored by the medical establishment. Furthermore, there is little dispute over the biochemical fact that zinc and manganese may replace copper and so reduce high copper levels. In evaluating the relative merits of the trace metals, then, we might categorize manganese as one of the "desirables" and copper as one of the "undesirables." This applies particularly to the schizophrenic.

In oral doses, manganese is never harmful, although in patients older than forty it has occasionally elevated blood pressure. The elevated pressure returns to normal when zinc alone is used.

Soil Depletion

Manganese is removed from the soil by current farming and food-processing practices. Soil erosion, leaching and soil exhaustion deplete the amount of manganese available to vegetables. Even normally manganese-rich foods are subject to wide variations. This depletion of the soil may be unsuspected since the foliage of plants may be lush without manganese. This is typified by the growth of lettuce. If lime is applied to solid clay, leafy vegetables grown in the more alkaline soil that is produced will contain much less manganese—simply because of the application of the lime. This finding points up the real need for scientific farming wherein the fertilizer will contain all of the trace elements in which the soil is deficient.

TABLE 3.1

**Selected foodstuffs with appreciable amounts
of manganese**

Mg per 100 gm edible parts

Cereals

Corn germ	10	Oats	3.0
Wheat bran	14	Corn flakes	0.04
Rice bran	26	White bread	0.25
Oat bran	10	Rice Krispies	1.0
Corn	1.0	Oatmeal	0.30-3.0
Wheat	5.0	Buckwheat	1.3
Rice	2.0		

Nuts

Walnuts	15	Pecans	1.5
Peanuts	1.9	Chestnuts	3.7

Spices

Cloves	30.0	Ginger	17.6
Cardamom	27.0		

Fruits

Strawberries	0.33	Prunes	0.08
Raspberries	0.12	Pineapple	0.1-3.0
Bananas	0.2-0.8	Cherries	0.03-0.78
Blueberries	0.15-1.9	Watermelon	0.03
Apples	0.20		

Vegetables

Lettuce	0.7-0.80	Onions	0.52-1.0
Spinach	0.2-15.0	Green beans	0.2-2.0
Peas	0.11	Dandelion greens	0.30
Lima beans	0.5-1.0	Carrots	0.06-0.6
Parsley	0.90-8.5		

Proteins

Meat	0.03	White	0.01
Whole egg	0.05	Sea fish	0.02
Shrimp	0.04	Fresh-water fish	0.06
Liver	0.12-0.53	Yolk	0.10
Clams	0.25	Snails	1.6

Miscellaneous

Yeast	0.53-0.90	Macaroni	0.5
Spaghetti	0.54	Coffee beans	2.0
Tea leaves	5-71	Egg noodles	0.78

Sources: D. Schlettwein-Gsell and S. Mommsen-Straub. *International Journal of Vitamin and Nutrition Research* 41:268, 1971, and A. Gormican. *Journal of the American Dietetic Association* 56:397, 1970.

Leafy vegetables and grains constitute our main sources of dietary manganese. The more alkaline the soil, the less manganese there will be in the leaves. This accounts for the variable range of manganese content. Liming of the soil increases foliage but decreases the manganese content. The germ or bran of the grain contains most manganese, but this is lost in the milling process. Note the drastic losses of manganese in corn: corn germ (10), corn (1) and corn flakes (0.04). Similarly drastic losses in manganese occur in the processing of wheat. Except for the organ meats (such as liver) protein is not a good source of manganese. Fish is low except for shellfish such as clams and snails. The daily requirement of man for manganese is about 4 mg.

References

Cook, D. G., et al. Chronic manganese intoxication. *Arch. Neurol.* 30:59, January 1974.

English, W. M. Report of the treatment with manganese chloride of 181 cases of schizophrenia, 33 of manic depression and 16 of other defects of psychoses at the Ontario Hospital, Brockville, Ontario. November 1929.

Everson, G. J. and Shrader, R. E. *J. of Nutr.* 94:89, 1968.

Hoskins, R. G. *J. Nerv. and Ment. Dis.* 79:59, 1934.

Hurley, L. S. Disproportionate growth in offspring of manganese deficient rats. *J. Nutrition* 74:274.

Kosenko, L. G. *Klin. Med.* 42:113, 1964.

Manganese for muscles and mother love. *Prevention*, p. 115, May 1969.

Manganese Update 1978

Manganese and the Brain

Manganese stimulates adenylate cyclase activity in brain and other tissues of the body as demonstrated in numerous experiments. In one study the striate cortex of rats was tested as a focus of manganese-catalyzed enzyme activity in this region of the brain. This study has great importance because cyclic-AMP plays a regulatory role in the action of several brain neurotransmitters. Thus, it was concluded that manganese has an important role in brain function.

In other studies, schizophrenic patients developed tardive dyskinesia, a Parkinson-like disease while on large doses of anti-schizophrenic medicines such as phenothiazine and butyrophenones and the newer drugs as well. Hair analysis done on patients who had ingested these drugs daily for several years revealed a manganese deficiency according to Dr. R. Kunin. High doses of a manganese chelate produced improvement in fourteen out of fifteen cases tested. Normally, high manganese concentrations are found in human basal ganglia where the ion is believed somehow to stimulate acetylcholine storage or activity. Manganese, acetylcholine and ATP are stored together as a complex in test tube experiments.

Our present knowledge of manganese function in human and animal brains cannot explain why a deficiency or intoxication of manganese results in Parkinson-like diseases.

Manganese and Blood Clotting

Manganese deficiency affects both man and animals. For example, it reduces the blood clotting response to extra vitamin K in chickens. One human patient with low clotting protein levels did not become normal until manganese supplements were given in addition to vitamin K. Manganese catalyzes the aggregation of human platelets in vitro. The manganese ion has an essential role in blood clotting and functions somewhere in the chain prior to direct vitamin K action.

Manganese and the Reproductive Function

Manganese-deficient female rats and chickens have defective ovulation and their offspring increased mortality. Deficient male rats and rabbits have a loss of libido, lack of semen and seminal tubule degeneration. The site of manganese action in the reproductive system is as yet unknown.

Manganese and Other Nutrients

The absorption of iron and manganese is inversely related. High iron in the diet inhibits manganese absorption, and, conversely, high manganese intake reduces iron absorption in several animal species, including man. This relationship also holds for calcium and zinc.

Calcium affects absorption and retention of manganese. In birds, high dietary levels of calcium phosphate aggravates manganese deficiency. In addition, manganese tested in the test tube at levels of 0.5 to 4.0 milli-molar concentration inhibits calcium-dependent histamine release. The inhibitory effect, however, is reversed by increased ion concentration. We know that both histadelic and histapenic patients do better if they have a daily source of zinc and manganese.

References

Evans, P. M. and Jones, B. M. Manganese induced aggregation of human platelets. *Cytobios* 13:37–44, 1975.

Foreman, J. C. and Morgan, J. L. The action of lanthanum and manganese on anaphylactic histamine secretion. *Br. J. Pharmac.* 48:527–537, 1973.

Kunin, R. A. Manganese and niacin in the treatment of drug-induced dyskinesias. *Orthomolecular Psychiatry* 5(1):a4–27, 1976.

Reuben, J. A ternary acetylcholine-manganese-ATP complex. *Febs Letters* 59(1):57–59, 1975.

Smeyers-velbeke, J., et al. Distribution of manganese in human brain tissue. *Clinica Chimerica Acta* 68:343–347, 1976.

Underwood, E. J. *Trace elements in human and animal nutrition.* New York: Academic Press, 1977, ch. 7.

CHAPTER 4

Sulfur: The Forgotten Essential Element

IN his comprehensive and recent book on trace elements in nutrition, E. J. Underwood does not discuss sulfur. (The two references to sulfur in his book are to its interaction with selenium.) Schroeder, in his several comments on sulfur as an essential element, indicates that for ordinary turnover in an adult body which contains a total of 140 gm, the daily requirement is 850 mg. Sulfur content is equalled by a potassium content (also 140 mg), and both sulfur and potassium content exceed that of sodium, which is only 100 gm. Yet we merrily salt our food each day, paying little heed to our sulfur and potassium needs.

The turnover of potassium and sodium is greater than that of sulfur. Both sulfur and potassium are found inside the cells, while sodium is found mainly outside the cells in the extracellular fluid. Every cell in the body contains sulfur, but the cells that contain the most are those of the skin, hair and joints. The horny layer of the skin, keratin, has a high content of sulfur as have the fingernails, toenails and hair. Sheep's wool and hair contain about 5 percent sulfur, and about 13 percent of sheep's wool is made up of the amino acid cystine. Since the curliness of hair depends on the sulfur-to-sulfur bonds of cystine, hair straighteners and curlers are designed to open up the S-to-S bonds and then set them in new arrangements, either straight-chain or curled-chain. If the waving solution is too strong or the hair too fine, the hair can be entirely dissolved instead of curled.

Peculiar odors in biology are usually due to sulfur compounds. The odor of burned hair or wool is no exception; this characteristic odor indicates the high sulfur content of hair.

Dietary Sulfur

Most of man's sulfur must come from food protein which provides four sulfur-containing amino acids—cysteine, cystine, taurine and methionine. The first three can be made in the body as long as adequate amounts of the essential amino acid methionine are contained in man's diet. Elemental sulfur will also allow the building of the first three amino aicds by the tissues of the body.

Vegetarians may become deficient in sulfur, particularly if they do not eat eggs. Many adults may be deficient in sulfur because of the misguided warnings against egg eating—our widespread cholesterol phobia. (Two eggs per day raise blood cholesterol by only 2 percent, which is not sufficient to cause atherosclerosis.)

Egg yolk is one of two foods that will darken a silver teaspoon. Since the other is red-hot peppers, most of us will choose the egg yolk as a source of our sulfur. For those who cannot eat eggs in any form (because of sensitivity), the local druggist will, on a physician's order, fill No. 1 capsules with flowers of sulfur. This dose, taken once each day, will provide one-quarter of the daily need, or 200 mg, of pure elemental sulfur. The other 600 mg can be obtained from the sulfur-containing amino acids. Even egg albumen or white of egg is higher in sulfur (1.62 percent) than casein from milk (0.80 percent) and soybean protein (0.38 percent). Muscle protein (as in beef) approaches egg white with 1.27 percent sulfur. Smelly foods such as onions and garlic contain appreciable amounts of sulfur. Indeed, the tear gas from sliced onions is a simple sulfur compound, and any blood-pressure-lowering effect of garlic is related to its "garlic" smell—one that is characteristic of an organic sulfur compound.

Cattle in feed lots lick on modern salt cakes made yellow with elemental sulfur. Chickens and pigs have sulfur added to their feed. Grandmother advocated sulfur and molasses each spring, and homeopathic physicians have continued to prescribe small doses of sulfur for many ailments. In early times some patients travelled to mineral springs or spas to drink regularly of the sulfur water, and even went so far as to bring home a jug of the medicinal waters for the rest of the family.

Sulfur water contains hydrogen sulfide. Ruminant animals such as sheep can make do with sulfur in the form of sulfate because the bacteria of their various stomachs will reduce the sulfate to sulfur. When man takes magnesium sulfate (Epsom salts) or sodium sulfate (horse physic), the sulfate is not absorbed but gathers water from the tissues and goes through the body with cathartic violence. When elemental sulfur was compared to sulfate sulfur in sheep (both at 0.5 percent level in the diet) either form produced better growth and better wool. The general dietary recommendation for sheep is for 0.2 percent elemental sulfur in the diet. The proper amount for man might be as little as 0.01 percent in cereal foods or a 100-mg scored tablet as a dietary supplement.

At present, dietary supplements containing sulfur are not available. One cannot give extra sulfur in the form of one of the amino acids since these often have adverse effects. For instance, methionine produces feelings of unreality. Simple organic sulfur compounds are not cleared for human use and all have a noticeable odor. One possible candidate for sulfur supplementation is the sulfur analogue of acetone called DMSO (dimethyl sulfoxide). This has the advantage of lipid solubility but has the disadvantage of being partially oxidized, so that the body may not be able to use it as a source of sulfur. Since DMSO is under careful clinical investigation, some answers may be forthcoming if the scientists remember to ask the crucial question:

does DMSO supply sulfur in a form usable by the body? The great lipid solubility of DMSO might get sulfur to the brain for the regrowth of nerves and treatment of epilepsy by allowing the brain to synthesize the stabilizing amino acid taurine.

Taurine and Epilepsy

Biochemical texts barely mention taurine; after all, it is not an essential sulfur amino acid like methionine. Taurine is a simple chemical with two carbon atoms separating a primary amino group and a sulfuric acid group. These chemical groups at both ends make taurine very water-soluble and thus hard to pass through the lipid membranes of the body. Taurine's function is to perch on cellular membranes, probably in neutralized form, and facilitate the passage of simple things such as the potassium and sodium ions and perhaps calcium or magnesium ions. Since taurine passes the blood-brain barrier very poorly, much of the brain taurine is probably built by the brain tissue.

Andre Barbeau, a dynamic physician at the Clinical Research Institute in Montreal, has studied taurine's role in animal and human epilepsy. The distribution of taurine in the human brain is similar to that of zinc and GABA (gamma-aminobutyric acid), both of which play an important calming role in nerve action. The injection of zinc in trace doses produced stretching and yawning in Barbeau's animals, as did GABA (which is monosodium glutamate with the one acid group removed). Because serum zinc is low and copper high in epileptics, Barbeau theorizes that seizures may occur when the zinc-to-copper ratio falls suddenly in the absence of adequate taurine, which cannot reach the brain easily and must be built in the brain. He believes that oral doses of taurine may help epileptics (but then, the other dietary forms of sulfur have not been tried—these are, of course, elemental sulfur or methionine or cysteine). We have found that elemental sulfur taken by mouth increases man's urinary taurine excretion.

Taurine is a stabilizer of membrane excitability and thus could control the onset of epileptic seizures. Taurine and sulfur could be factors in the control of many disorders, including the known biochemical changes in the aging process. Disorders of the skin and nails might improve with added sulfur in our diet. (In 1899, the *Journal of the American Medical Association* published an article on the use of sulfur in psoriasis.)

Previous Uses of Sulfur in Therapeutics

In the nineteenth century, elemental sulfur was used to treat many disorders because no better remedies were available. If these uses are reviewed with the thought that sulfur deficiency may perhaps occur in man as well as in animals, then some of the old uses of sulfur make good sense.

Psoriasis is a scaly condition of the skin which, in mild cases, occurs on the elbows and knees or behind the belt buckle—i.e., at pressure points. The scales may disappear in summer with sunlight, but return quickly in winter. Large doses of zinc are helpful, and small oral doses of sulfur may also help. The normal formation of melanin pigment requires two amino acids and sulfur plus sunlight. Nutrients which help the skin to tan (pigmenting process) should help psoriasis. These would be adequate protein, vitamin B-6, zinc and sulfur. Patients with psoriasis are more likely than others to get arthritis or joint diseases.

Rheumatoid arthritis patients seem, as a rule, to dislike eggs—at present, our only good source of sulfur. Since yolks turned grandmother's silver spoons black (because of silver sulfide) grandma had special little bone spoons for eating soft-boiled eggs long before the fad of throwing plastic spoons away. In the 1920s, colloidal sulfur was given intravenously or intramuscularly to arthritic patients without adequate control as to the possible benefit. Sulfur in oil was also given in both arthritic and mental patients. The joints are high in sulfate-containing compounds. The most common is chondroitin sulfate of the cartilages. All patients with rheumatoid arthritis would do well to eat at least two eggs per day to provide adequate sulfur for their needs.

The use of sulfur in large doses as a laxative dates back to antiquity. With bacterial action, hydrogen sulfide is formed in the intestine and (as with most intestinal gas) is absorbed. The local hydrogen sulfide is reported to promote peristalsis of the large bowel and facilitate daily bowel movements. Modern studies on sulfur as a laxative have yet to be done. Hydrogen sulfide was thought to be useful in heavy metal poisoning, but here again, modern data are not available. (The sulfur and molasses of grandma's day was probably given for the laxative effect.)

The physician frequently wishes to normalize the flora of the intestine after antibiotic therapy. Acidophilus tablets or buttermilk is sometimes suggested. Certainly egg yolks, with their high sulfur content, or elemental sulfur could be used to normalize the flora or change an unwelcome yeast or fungal flora.

Lack of Sulfur in Soil

The soil in many areas of the world is deficient in sulfur. The glaciated areas are known to have lost sulfur, selenium, iodide and zinc. Commercial fertilizers seldom restore these trace elements to the soil. Plants depend on the soil for sulfur in the form of the sulfate ion. This is taken into the plant, where enzymes convert the sulfate into the many organic sulfur compounds which both plants and animals need. In most instances, the major sources of animal dietary sulfur are the two amino acids, methionine and cysteine. From these the body builds the essential compounds coenzyme A, heparin, glutathione, lipoic acid and biotin. The flora of the world build with sulfur the various penicillins and the characteristic odors of garlic, onion and mustard—not to mention horseradish.

References

Barbeau, A. and Donaldson, J. Zinc, taurine and epilepsy. *Arch. Neurol.* 30:52, 1974.

Martin, W. G. The neglected nutrient sulphur. *The Sulphur Institute Journal* p. 5, Spring 1968.

Math, O. H. and Oldfield, J. E. *Symposium sulfur in nutrition.* Westport, Connecticut: The AVI Publishing Co., 1970.

Schroeder, H. A. *The trace elements and man.* Old Greenwich, Connecticut: Devin-Adair, 1973.

Shohl, A. T. *Sulfur in mineral metabolism.* chap. 8. New York: Reinhold Publishing Co., 1939.

Underwood, E. J. *Trace elements in human and animal nutrition.* 3rd ed. New York: Academic Press, 1971.

Van Gelder, N. M. Antagonism by taurine of cobalt induced epilepsy in cat and mouse. *Brain Research* 47:157, 1972.

Sulfur Update 1978

Onions and Garlic

Nutritionists and doctors are beginning to re-emphasize the importance of garlic and onions in health care, for these sulfur-containing foods may be important sources of reduced sulfur in the body. They alleviate various disorders of the stomach, circulatory system and sinuses, and theoretically, such sulfur compounds should help remove our body burden of heavy metals such as copper, cadmium, mercury and lead.

Throughout history garlic has been said to have medicinal properties. Since World War I, extensive research has been carried out on garlic in many regions of the world, partly as a result of its successful use as an antiseptic in the prevention and treatment of gangrene and other serious infections. Garlic also helps control pus formation. In addition, the growth of Mycobacterium tuberculosis, Staphyococcus aureus and

Brucella abortus is inhibited by a garlic juice concentration of 0.02 percent or by application of garlic paste. The anti-bacterial effect of garlic has been attributed to allicin (Table 4.1).

TABLE 4.1

Sulfur Scents

Onion =	$CH_3CH_2CH = S = O$ (Tear gas)
Onion	$CH_3CH_2CH_2$-S-S-CH_2CH_2-CH_3 (Flavor)
	$CH_3CH_2CH_2$-S-S-$CH_2CH_2 = CH_2$ (APDS)
Garlic =	H_3C-S-S-CH_3
Garlic (Allicin)	$CH_2 = CH\ CH_2\ S$-S-$CH_2CH = CH_2$

$$\underset{\underset{CH_2 = CH\ CH_2\ S-CH_2CH\ COOH}{|}}{NH_2}$$

Garlic (Allium)

$$\overset{O\ H_2\ H\ \ H}{\underset{H_3C - S - S - C - C = C - CH_3}{||\ \ |\ \ |\ \ \ |}}$$

Skunk = 1) Odors

$$\overset{H_2\ H\ \ H}{\underset{2)\ HS - C - C = C - CH_3}{|\ \ |\ \ \ |}}$$

$$\overset{H}{\underset{3)\ HS - C - C - C - CH_3}{\underset{|\ \ \ \ |\ \ \ \ |}{CH_3 - H_2 - H_2}}}$$

Asparagus urinary odors are caused by:

$$\overset{O}{\underset{CH_2 = CH - C - S - CH_3}{||}}$$

$$\overset{O}{\underset{CH_3 = SCH_2CH_2 - C - S - CH_3}{||}}$$

The original compound in asparagus is odorless and has not yet been identified.

Garlic lowers high blood pressure and may protect against increased serum cholesterol and arteriosclerosis. In one study, ten healthy young volunteers fed four slices of bread with 3½ ounces of butter had a sharp rise of cholesterol levels within four hours. When garlic, either raw or cooked, was consumed with the fatty meal, cholesterol levels stayed low. Garlic also slows blood coagulation time because it causes blood platelets not to clump together as quickly. For hemophiliacs this would be dangerous, but for the majority of people whose blood clots too quickly garlic could be helpful.

Garlic promotes free breathing and as an expectorant clears up mucous congestions. In one study, a solution of garlic oil administered as 10 to 25 nose drops cleared up the congested nostrils of a large group of patients within thirteen to twenty minutes. Garlic pills (with the active ingredient allicin) have been successful in treating diarrhea, nausea, gas, nervous stomach and belching.

The onion has many properties similar to those of garlic. Onions slow blood coagulation and prevent a rise in serum cholesterol when ingested with a high-fat meal. The onion also has a hypoglycemic effect. Administering APDS (see Table 4.1) to diabetic rabbits reduced their insulin requirement. A dosage of 0.123 g/kg body weight taken by six fasting normal volunteers resulted in a fall in blood glucose levels and a rise in serum insulin. Onions, whether boiled, fried or as a juice extracted from crushed bulbs, all have the same beneficial effects because the sulfur compounds are relatively water insoluble.

The effects of garlic extend to other members of the genus Allium—leeks, chives and shallots—but to a lesser degree. Thus far, the beneficial effects of all these foods can be attributed to the detoxification of the sulfur compounds.

Asparagus also provides simple sulfur compounds which, when excreted in the urine, provide the typical odor.

We should not depend on proteins for our sulfur

compounds when nature has provided numerous vegetables with appreciable sulfur content.

References

Augusti, K. J. Effect on alloin diabetes of allyl propyl disulphide obtained from onion. *Comica Chimica Act A* 61:172–173, 1974.

Augusti, K. T. and Benaim, M. E. Effect of essential oil of onion (allyl propyl disulphide) on blood glucose, free fatty acid and insulin levels of normal subjects. *Comica Chimica Acta* 60:121–123, 1975.

Bogin, E. and Abrams, M. The effect of garlic extract on the activity of some enzymes. *Fd. Cosmet. Toxicol.* 14:417–419, 1976.

Clark, M. Garlic, the pungent health protector. *Prevention* 1, 1977, pp. 163–168.

Gottlieb, B. Break a cold's grip with dietary fire. *Prevention* 10, 1976, pp. 107–110.

Harris, C. J. *The book of garlic*. San Francisco: Panjandum Press, 1975.

The herbs and the heart. *Nutrition Reviews* 34(2):43–44, 1976.

Kinderlehrer, J. Good for your appetite, great for your circulation. *Prevention* 5, 1976, pp. 118–126.

Put onions in your garden this year. *Prevention* 4, 1977, pp. 144–147.

Roueche, B. A friend in disguise: garlic. *New Yorker*, 28 October 1974, pp. 55–62.

White, R. H. Occurrence of S-methyl thioesters in urines of humans after they have eaten asparagus. *Science* 189:417–419, 1976.

CHAPTER 5

Selenium:
Stepchild of Sulfur

SELENIUM, occurring naturally as either a red powder or a gray crystal, is among the most poisonous elements in the universe; and yet, in pure form, it is an essential trace mineral for animals and man. It is a by-product of copper refining and is used in the manufacture of photoelectric equipment, in paints and in xerography. It is widely but unevenly distributed in the earth's crust. South Dakota's soil is very high while Ohio's is very low.

Selenium-rich soils are thought to result from ancient volcanic eruptions and subsequent leaching to ancient inland seas long since evaporated. Wind and rain may remove selenium from the soil into the sea, thus causing a deficiency in locally grown plants and animal feed. Areas which were glaciated in the ice age have had all of the selenium removed by slow-melting glaciers. This action also removed zinc, sulfur and iodine from the soil. The wheat and corn grown in Ohio are so low in selenium that cattle feed was, at one time, shipped from South Dakota in order to supply adequate selenium. The United States Department of Agriculture now allows the fortification of animal feeds with trace amounts of selenium.

However, too much selenium in the soil—as in South Dakota—produces toxicity and occasionally death in ruminant animals. Selenium also occurs as a water contaminant around heavily irrigated land. The animal feeds of South Dakota must be diluted with forage grown elsewhere. An adequate dietary intake of selenium for animals is 200 parts per billion (ppb). This level would probably suffice for man also.

Too much selenium, generally absorbed from inorganic salts or from organic compounds in plants, produces toxic symptoms. These include loss of hair, nails and teeth; dermatitis; lassitude and progressive paralysis. Acute poisoning causes fever (103° to 105°), increased respiratory and capillary rate, gastroenteritis, myelitis (inflammation of the spinal cord and bone marrow), anorexia and even death.

Selenium also has some important beneficial effects. It protects against the toxic effects of the pollutant cadmium. Tests on laboratory animals have shown that it also protects against high-mercury tuna fish. In humans, it increases the effectiveness of vitamin E, and it appears to reduce the chances of all types of cancer. Selenium is an antioxidant that helps prevent chromosome breakage in tissue culture. Damaged chromosomes cause not only birth defects but also cancer if the damage to the DNA (found in the cells' nuclei) disturbs the inhibitors that control the cells' tendency to multiply. Studies have shown that in communities where selenium intake is low, the cancer rate is high.

Amount in the Human Blood

Rhead et al. in California have analyzed human blood and found detectable levels in every fraction tested. Hemoglobin has 0.65 ppm, alpha-2 globulins 5.76 ppm, transferrin 3.4 ppm, and ceruloplasm 5.4 ppm. Insulin, which is known to contain much sulfur, has 4.0 ppm of selenium. In these instances selenium may occur as a contaminant of sulfur. In one enzyme, glutathione peroxidase, however, selenium is the only active trace element. The study of the levels of this enzyme in mental disease and also cancer would be most worthwhile.

Males seem to have a higher requirement for selenium than females. Most infants who die are males. Of the thirty-five thousand infant deaths per year in the United States, about one-quarter are associated with selenium and/or vitamin E deficiency. Almost none of these babies is breast fed, and it is significant that human milk contains up to six times as much selenium as cow's milk and twice as much vitamin E. Also, some children suffering from malnutrition fail to grow when given a recuperative diet unless selenium is added. Australian investigators have suggested that selenium deficiency may be involved in sudden and unexplained crib deaths. Selenium is necessary for protein synthesis; thus, its importance cannot be ignored.

One disadvantage of selenium, however, is its possible tendency to increase dental caries in children up to the age of ten. Trace elements may alter susceptibility to caries by changing the chemical composition of the dental enamel during the period of tooth formation. Heavy consumption of selenium seems to decrease the beneficial effect of fluoride, which helps prevent tooth decay. However, ethical considerations have prevented the carrying out of experiments on human subjects.

Food Sources

Good food sources of selenium include brewer's yeast, garlic, liver and eggs. Foods from animal sources are generally richer in the mineral than those from vegetable sources, so vegetarians should supplement their diet with brewer's yeast tablets to fulfill the requirement. Unfortunately, all foods lose selenium in processing— for example, brown rice has fifteen times the selenium content of white rice, and whole-wheat bread contains twice as much selenium as white bread. It is to be hoped that in future the government will encourage the addition of selenium to staple foods with the goal of preventing deficiency and further reducing the cancer rate in this country.

References

Hadjimarkos, D. M. Selenium in relation to dental caries. *Fd. Cosmet. Toxicol.* 11:1083–1095, 1973.

Harr, J. R. and Muth, O. H. Selenium poisoning in domestic animals and its relationship to man. *Clinical Toxicology* 5(2):175–186, 1972.

Rhead, W. J. et al. Selenium in human plasma: levels in blood proteins and behavior upon dialysis acidification and reduction. *Bioinorganic Chemistry* 3:217–223, 1974.

Selenium Update 1978

For Growth

Selenium deficiency has been directly related to several animal diseases: nutritional muscular dystrophy, exudative diathesis (spontaneous swelling and hemorrhages), pancreatic atrophy, liver necrosis and infertility. A dietary selenium supplement, 10-100 ppb, was found to increase the growth rate of selenium-depleted rats fed diets containing adequate levels of vitamin E. Selenium is required for growth in human cells in culture and may be necessary for normal growth.

Cancer

Human mortality from cancer of the stomach, esophagus and rectum has particularly increased in low-selenium areas of the country. Cancer death rates are smaller for cancer of the small and large intestine, pharnyx, bladder and kidney. The difference between low-selenium and high-selenium areas is insignificant for cancer of the lung, pancreas, prostate, lymphatics and leukemia. Whether low selenium in the blood exists before the cancer develops or as a consequence of it is unknown. In addition, measuring blood levels is a generally poor way to test for a deficiency. Selenium appears to be stored in the liver, and blood levels remain constant until these stores are depleted. Hair tests may prove diagnostically superior.

Glutathione Peroxidase—A Unique Enzyme Containing Selenium

Glutathione peroxidase, a tripeptide enzyme containing selenium, catalyzes the removal of hydrogen peroxide, an oxidizer. Glutathione peroxidase destroys peroxides before they can attack cellular membranes, while vitamin E acts within the membrane itself preventing the oxidation of membrane lipids. If peroxides can trigger cancer, then glutathione peroxidase may prevent cancer. The activity of this enzyme varies with species, tissue and amount of selenium in the diet. While some scientists suggest that glutathione peroxidase activity is genetically inherited, the majority feel that peroxidase activity represents overall selenium status of the organism. Several cases of anemia in premature infants have been attributed to reduced glutathione activity in erythrocytes.

The effect of peroxides on lens tissue has not been identified conclusively. Peroxides are likely to cause the oxidation of protein components and membrane lipids, both of which have been related to cataract formation. Normally, the selenium concentration increases fourfold in normal human lenses between birth and age eighty-five, while in cataract lenses the selenium concentration is less than one-sixth that of normal lenses compared to the same age group. Men have large stores of selenium in the testicles and secrete it in the seminal fluid.

Selenium Supplements and Health

Besides cadmium, selenium is also an antagonist of poisonous arsenic, silver, mercury and copper; it can reduce the toxicity of these elements and the reverse is also true. Selenosis is rare in humans but may become more common as a result of the widespread use of xerography machines. These machines contain selenium plates and emit a form of selenium in the air. Hence, toxicity could result from long-term close exposure to a machine that runs all day. Selenium sulfide is an ingredient in dandruff shampoos but presents no potential hazard because the compound is insoluble.

In laboratory tests on animals, various selenium forms were tried: natural selenium, se-methionine, se-cystine, mono and dicarboxcyclic acids or selenites. In hens, natural selenium was preferable but other animal tests gave different results. Brewer's yeast is a good source of selenium, but the best selenium compound for humans remains an important research problem.

Evidence is mounting that while selenium does not substitute for sulfur in the human body, it has entirely unique biochemical functions.

References

Chemical and Engineering News, 3 May 1976, pp. 24–25.

Gross, S. Hemolytic anemia in premature infants: relationship to vitamin E, selenium, gluthathione peroxidase and erthocyte lipids. *Seminars in Hematology* 13(3):187–199, 1975.

Harkin, J. M., et al. Elevation of selenium levels by xerography. Personal communication.

Hill, L. H. Interrelationships of selenium with other trace elements. *Fed. Proc.* 34(11):2096–2100, 1975.

Hookstra, W. G. Biochemical function of selenium and its relation to vitamin E. *Fed. Proc.* 34:2083–2089, 1975.

Mckeehan, W. C., et al. Selenium is an essential trace nutrient for growth of WI-38 diploid human fibroblasts. *Proc. Natl. Acad. Sci.* 73(6):2023–2027, 1976.

Prasad, A. S. *Trace elements in human health and disease.* New York: Academic Press, 1976, Vol. 2, Ch. 30–32.

Underwood, E. J. *Trace elements in human and animal nutrition.* New York: Academic Press, 1977, Ch. 12.

CHAPTER 6

Calcium
and Demineralization

EVERY school child knows that the mineral calcium is necessary for strong bones and teeth. In fact, 99 percent of the calcium in the body is found in the bones. The other 1 percent is just as vital because it is involved in controlling blood clotting mechanisms, the excitability of nerves and muscles, the function of parathyroid hormone and the action of vitamin D.

Calcium occurs in the blood, the fluid surrounding cells, cell membranes and intracellular organelles. Unfortunately, according to a survey released in 1968 by the USDA, over 30 percent of the human population of this nation is calcium deficient. Calcium is of further interest in mental disease since intravenous injections were used in the early 1930s to produce lucid intervals in some schizophrenics. Those patients who responded may have been the histadelic or high-histamine type, since only one out of five patients responded. Calcium ion is a histamine-releasing agent.

What Is Calcium Deficiency?

Without calcium, muscles cannot contract. Deficiency causes increased irritability, osteoporosis (softening of the bones), osteomalacia (another type of bone-softening disease) and rickets. According to Leo Lutwak, Professor of Medicine at the School of Medicine, University of California at Los Angeles, "Various surveys have indicated that approximately 30 percent of women over the age of 55 and men over the age of 60 have had sufficient mineral loss to have produced at least one fracture."

The bone-softening disease cannot be detected reliably by X rays until 30 percent or more of the bone mineral has been lost. Unfortunately, in Dr. Lutwak's opinion, his studies suggest that once vertebral fracture has occurred, the progression of softening of the bones cannot be stopped. Other researchers disagree, and some suggest that fluoride in addition to calcium might be more helpful than calcium alone.

Loss of Calcium with Bed Rest or Space Flights

Bed rest is bad for human physiology since calcium is lost from bones and nitrogen is lost from muscles. In the confinement of their spaceship the astronauts in their eight-day space mission lost 200 mg of calcium per day in spite of a daily routine of vigorous exercises. The absence of gravity in space makes walking impossible, so that the bones start to lose calcium from inactivity, and continue to do so. More ingenious elastic apparatus is needed to exercise the big muscles of the legs and back.

Going to bed with a cold or minor misery may impair health because of this calcium and nitrogen loss. With serious illness some bed rest may be necessary at the start, but the resourceful individual will start exercising after the fever breaks or the heart pain stops. Otherwise, the road back from absolute bed rest will be a long and weary one.

For example, on the sixth day after a severe heart attack most individuals can start finger exercises, the next day arm exercises and the tenth day leg exercises while still in bed. Unless this type of exercise program is initiated, always on the advice of the doctor, the bright day will dawn when the doctor says, "Now you may get out of bed," and the patient experiences rubbery knees and even invalidism because of inactivity.

Extra Calcium Tablets Require Extra Zinc

We know from numerous animal studies that extra calcium in the diet decreases zinc absorption. Most animals are on a high-cereal diet which contains considerable phytate. Calcium phytate chelates (nabs onto) zinc ions so that they are lost from the body. Since older patients usually need both zinc and calcium, these should be separated. Even inositol should be separated in time from the zinc and calcium so that maximum absorption of both calcium and zinc are effected.

Hypoglycemics on High-protein Diets Require More Calcium

Drs. Bekha and Linbowiler at the University of Wisconsin have studied young men on a standard calcium intake of 500 mg per day. When the protein intake was 47 gm per day, calcium retention was 31 mg. At 92 gm of protein per day, retention was *minus* 58 mg and—even worse—*minus* 120 mg at 142 gm, with none of the nine subjects in calcium balance. The fecal excretion of calcium was not affected, so the great loss of calcium was all by the urinary pathway. The calcium loss can be overcome by extra calcium in the diet. Older patients on a high-protein diet develop osteoporosis while older vegetarians do not. The acid ash of the protein is responsible for the calcium loss. Obviously, hypoglycemic patients on high protein diets need bone meal or dolomitic calcium tablets twice a day.

Calcium Levels and Psychiatric Depression

Dr. F. F. Flach of Cornell Medical Center has pioneered the study of calcium balance in psychiatric depression. Effective treatment of the depression lowers the blood serum calcium level and increases the retention of calcium by the body. Patients with lack of response to treatment do not show this shift in calcium metabolism. These authors relate the calcium shift to adrenalin-like neuro-humors which might relieve depression.

Dr. John S. Carman has a similar idea involving the urinary excretion of calcium and magnesium. Patients placed on lithium therapy may show a high serum level of both calcium and magnesium. If their depression is lifted by the lithium therapy, the serum blood levels will decrease and urinary excretion of these two elements increase. Carman and his colleagues propose this as a test for the antidepressant response to lithium and other drugs.

What Amounts of Calcium Are Needed in the Body?

The National Academy of Sciences states that men, women and children (aged 1 to 10) need 800 mg of calcium daily. Infants need only 360 to 540 mg, while older boys and girls and pregnant and lactating women need 1200 mg daily. Dr. Lutwak believes 1000 mg of calcium daily in older people may completely prevent osteoporosis.

Regardless of age, whether a person is ingesting adequate calcium or not, the body will lose this mineral every day. Approximately 100 to 200 mg of calcium is filtered from the blood and excreted in the urine. An additional 125 to 180 mg is excreted in the digestive juices, remains unabsorbed and passes out of the body in the feces. Also, a small amount is lost in sweat. Ingesting 380 mg of calcium daily will *not* prevent the bones from wasting away. For example, if a woman at the age of twenty consumed only 380 mg of calcium per day, she would probably have lost two-thirds of the calcium in her body by the age of fifty. As aging occurs, the body's absorption of calcium becomes less efficient. Also, excitement or depressive emotional states can markedly increase calcium loss.

Like most other substances, an excess of calcium may produce undesirable results. If an excess of calcium is added to blood plasma, it prevents coagulation. Nervous and muscular functions can be depressed by overly large quantities of calcium. Children receiving an excess of vitamin D take up too much calcium and may have stomach upsets and retarded growth. However, since a sizeable portion of the population suffers from calcium deficiency, hypercalcemia (excess calcium) is a rare problem by comparison.

Calcium is essential, but its interaction with other vitamins and minerals must not be overlooked. A lack of magnesium can cause calcium deposits in muscles, heart and kidney. This results in kidney stones. The use of enough vitamin B-6 to produce recall of nightly dreams will allow enough pyridoxic acid to form to prevent kidney stones of the calcium oxalate type. Many urologists put their stone-forming patients on some vitamin B-6, but real success depends on a dose adequate to ensure that some goes over into the urine as pyridoxic acid. In hyperparathyroidism, calcium is mobilized from the bones excessively. Patients with this condition may also have kidney stones, but the removal of the enlarged parathyroid gland provides prompt relief.

Calcium in the Histadelic Patient

The Brain Bio Center introduced the use of calcium gluconate 500 mg A.M. and P.M. for the treatment of the histadelic patient (high blood histamine). Calcium ions have a histamine-releasing effect so that when given with Dilantin and methionine the blood histamine level is reduced. In the treatment of 100 histadelic patients with calcium gluconate 1 gm per day only 2 cases of kidney gravel were encountered—in both instances in female patients. Because of this, we usually recommend only one tablet of calcium gluconate per day in smaller histadelic females.

Good Sources of Calcium

Milk is ordinarily the best source of a balanced solution of calcium, magnesium and phosphorus. Two glasses of milk per day should be drunk by every growing individual and every pregnant woman. One 8-ounce glass per day should be drunk by every adult, and if this rule is followed then the adult will not lose the ability to burn lactose or milk sugar. Twenty percent of white adults and 80 percent of black adults cannot digest lactose, mainly because they stopped using milk in early adulthood.

One 8-ounce glass of whole milk supplies 30 percent of the daily calcium requirement. This glass of milk has 160 calories, while skim milk has only 90 calories and contains all of the calcium, magnesium and phosphate of whole milk. The color of skim milk can be improved by stirring in the yolk of an egg, which adds almost 5 percent of the daily need for calcium. The glass of milk also provides 25 percent of the daily need for riboflavin (vitamin B-2). Cheese (made from milk) is another good source of calcium.

Dolomitic calcium and magnesium can be used by the adult who is sensitive to milk. Since the magnesium makes the calcium soluble, the danger of kidney stones which occurs with calcium alone is eliminated. Two 300 mg tablets A.M. and P.M. are sufficient.

Bone meal provides calcium and magnesium and other minerals such as fluoride as they occur in our well-fed animals. Since the fluoride content may not be sufficient to prevent osteoporosis in older people, some should have a daily sodium fluoride tablet in addition.

The eggshell—usually thrown out—is a splendid source of calcium and trace elements. Eggshells can be used to sweeten vinegar and lemon juice by neutralizing the acid, so that sugar is not needed. Salad dressings made from vinegar or lemon juice neutralized with egg shells need no sugar. Eggs allowed to stand for twenty-four hours in either cider or wine vinegar will have a soft shell. The whole egg can then be thrown into the blender to make an eggnog. (So-called white vinegar is only diluted acetic acid and should be avoided.) The eggshells, ordinarily too gritty to eat, can thus be recycled to fill human calcium needs. When eggshells are used to sweeten cider or wine vinegar, the calcium is then in the vinegar as calcium acetate. Since the vinegar is less sour and is now loaded with natural trace elements, it will be more nutritious when used in salads or to make home-made mayonnaise.

Calcium nutrition is a complex matter which must be regarded as a whole rather than discussed in a fragmentary manner. Dr. William Strain of Cleveland has stated that trace element nutriture is like a giant spider web; if one branch of the web is pulled, the whole web of trace elements becomes distorted. Calcium balance, so closely related to magnesium, zinc, iron, selenium and sulfur balance, exemplifies this analogy very well.

References

Adams, R. and Murray, F. *Minerals: Kill or cure?* New York: Larchmont Books, 1974.

Flach, F. F. Calcium metabolism in states of depression. *Brit. J. Psychiat.* 110:588–593, 1964.

Flach, F. F. and Faragalla, F. F. The effects of imipramine and electro-convulsive therapy on the excretion of various minerals in depressed patients. *Brit. J. Psychiat.* 116:437–438, 1970.

Lutwak, L. Continuing need for dietary calcium through life. *Geriatrics* 29, 1974.

Robinson, C. H. *Fundamentals of normal nutrition.* New York: Macmillan, 1973.

Sollmann. *A manual of pharmacology.* Philadelphia: W. B. Saunders, 1957.

Trager, J. *The bellybook.* New York: Grossman, 1972.

Calcium Update 1978

More than one-third of tested renal patients on dialysis (these patients had many nutritional complications) had severe calcification of the heart, lungs, stomach or kidneys. Calcification of soft tissue was reported to progress during dialysis therapy. The cardiac deaths of six dialysis patients (on dialysis for six months or more) were directly related to calcification of heart muscles and/or the conduction system. The correlation of dialysis duration to degree of calcification was not absolute; clearly, other nutritional factors are involved. The nature of the phosphorus-binding gels used in most treatments of renal patients is usually aluminum hydroxide.

Calcium deficiency is marked by increased nervousness and bone weakness. Osteomalacia has been associated with use of anti-convulsants which are antifolate and also accelerate the breakdown of vitamin D. A vitamin D deficiency results in impaired calcium absorption. For example, calcium-deficient mothers give birth to children with reduced bone density. A deficiency in calcium also plays an important role in cardiac arrythmias. Calcium is functionally important for many cardiac cells and is primarily responsible for generation of the electrical potential in the conducting system.

Hyperoxaluria is a cause of calcium oxalate kidney stones and usually results from excess oxalate in the diet. Normally, small amounts of oxalate in the diet binds with calcium and precipitates from solution in the intestine. The bound product is then excreted in the stool. When calcium or zinc supplements are added to the diet, the amount of oxalate in the urine is reduced and almost all the supplemental calcium is excreted in the stool.

Calcium supplements such as bone meal, dolomite, calcium lactate or milk are good and healthy ways to promote sleep.

References

Calcium treatment may prevent formation of kidney stones. *Internal Medicine* 2(7):4, 1976.

Krishnamachari, K.A.V.R. and Iyenger, L. Effect of maternal malnutrition on the bone density of the neonates. *Am. J. Clin. Nutrition* 28:482–486, 1975.

Reunanen, M. I., et al. Serum calcium balance during early phase of diphenyldantoin therapy. *Int. J. Clin. Pharmacol.* 14(1):15–19, 1976.

Some advances in cardiac research. *JAMA* 235(14):1411–1418, 1976.

CHAPTER 7

Phosphate Update 1978

THE story goes that a male worker in an acid plant disappeared while at work. After investigating the circumstances surrounding his disappearance, his wife concluded that he must have fallen into one of the hot acid vats and been consumed. She consulted a pharmacologist who promptly got a court order to have each of the acid vats analyzed for phosphoric acid and calcium. All vats were found to have traces of each element, but one vat had the equivalent of 1 kgm (2 pounds) of phosphorus and 1 kgm (2 pounds) of calcium added to the acid. These two inorganic elements are the most plentiful in the human body and could only have been present in that amount if a human body had fallen into the vat. The insurance company paid the death claim, and burial of the remains was not a problem since the man had requested in his will that he be cremated!

The two pound load of phosphorus in the human body is not in the bones alone but in all other tissues as well. Phosphate functions as the body's major anion, while calcium, magnesium, potassium and sodium are the major cations. Phosphate deficiency upsets the normal balance between phosphate, magnesium, calcium and potassium. Like calcium, most phosphorus is stored in the skeletal system; therefore, the concentration of phosphate influences the uptake and distribution of calcium. In a rare case of hypercalcemia, phosphate administered intravenously quickly lowered serum calcium concentrations. Phosphate mobilizes calcium from the extracellular fluid into the bone.

Phosphorus exists in the body as inorganic and organic phosphates. The concentration of phosphates in serum decreases with age, the normal values for children being 4.0 to 7.1 mg percent and for adults 2.7 to 4.5 mg percent. Lowered blood phosphate, hypophosphatemia, may result from alcoholism, antacid therapy, intravenous glucose, barbiturate therapy, pregnancy and vitamin D deficiency. The clinical symptoms of phosphate deficiency are muscle weakness (to the point of respiratory arrest), anemia and increased susceptibility to infection. Anemia results from an alteration in red blood cell membranes. Decreased resistance to infection is related to lowered activity of white blood cells which results from phosphate deficiency. (For a list of foods rich in phosphate, see Table 7.1.)

TABLE 7.1

Foods rich in phosphate (mg/100 gm)

Brewer's yeast	2500
Rice bran	1400
Wheat bran	1300
Pumpkin seeds, wheat germ	1100
Sunflower seeds	800
Sesame seeds, soybeans	600
Almond, bran flakes, liver	500
Cowpeas, peanuts, kidney beans, lentils	400
Flounder, mung beans, chickpeas, chicken	200
Eggs, beef	300

Both hypomagnesemia and hypokalemia (low potassium) have been associated with phosphorus deficiency. The primary cause cannot be identified with complete certainty. Excessive excretion of phosphate and potassium can result from magnesium deficiency.

Similarily, potassium and phosphate influence retention and absorption of magnesium.

Treatment of Hypophosphatemia

For emaciated individuals, oral feeding of skim milk or low-fat milk is useful because each quart of milk contains approximately 1.0 grams of calcium and phosphorus. Amino acid-supplemented skim milk is easily tolerated when whole milk causes gas and diarrhea.

A mixture of sodium hydrogen phosphate and sodium di-hydrogen phosphate may be used orally as a phosphate supplement and is available over the counter at any local pharmacy. A mixture of potassium di-hydrogen phosphate is available for addition to intravenous fluids.

The best means of adding supplemental phosphate to the diet is through a combination of bone meal and dolomite morning and night. Bone meal provides adequate phosphate and dolomite provides the magnesium necessary for absorption.

References

Adams, R. and Murray, F. *Minerals: Kill or cure?* New York: Larchmont Books, 1974, pp. 76–86.

Knochel, J. P. The pathophysiology and clinical characteristics of severe hypophosphatemia. *Arch. Intern. Med.* 137:203–220, 1977.

Moser, C. R. and Fessel, J. W. Rheumatic manifestation of hypophosphatemia. *Arch. Intern. Med.* 134:674–678, 1974.

Rude, R. K. and Singer, F. R. When dietary phosphate is not enough. *Drug Therapy*, August 1976, pp. 114–118.

CHAPTER 8

Magnesium

MAGNESIUM derives its name from the Greek city Magnesia, where large deposits of magnesium carbonate were found. The first record of the medical use of magnesium dates back to the Italian Renaissance when salts of magnesium were used as a laxative. Today magnesium is used in Epsom salts (magnesium sulfate) and milk of magnesia (suspended magnesium hydroxide) because of its laxative properties.

Magnesium is a mineral essential to most living things and is found in abundance in man. Because of the large quantity in the body, magnesium is termed a bulk or major element rather than a trace element. Humans need magnesium for the production and transfer of energy, muscle contraction, protein synthesis and nerve excitability. Magnesium functions as a co-factor, assisting enzymes in catalyzing many chemical reactions.

Can I Have Too Much Magnesium?

An excess of magnesium can be toxic, but magnesium intoxication is rare, occurring only if the body experiences an unusual decrease in urinary excretion or a great increase in absorption and sometimes after intramuscular injection. Certain types of bone tumors and cancer in women may also raise the magnesium in the plasma to high levels. Hypermagnesia (excess magnesium) can cause depression of the central nervous system (it has been used for anesthesia), and an extreme excess of magnesium can cause death. Magnesium intoxication, however, is almost unknown.

Can I Be Magnesium Deficient?

Magnesium deficiencies are found in chronic alcoholism, cirrhosis of the liver, diabetic acidosis and various other illnesses. Patients who are fed magnesium-free fluids intravenously often become deficient.

Hypomagnesia (lowered blood magnesium) occurs in arteriosclerosis (degeneration of the arteries) and may lead to disturbances of heart rhythm. Dr. Janos Rigo of Semmelweis Medical University, Budapest, found that a high-magnesium diet lowered blood pressure and prevented "precocious aging" of the aorta in rats with experimentally induced hypertension.

Everyone is apt to become magnesium deficient, since the mineral is stripped from many of our foods through processing. Wheat loses almost all magnesium through refining, and refined sugars and fats contain almost no magnesium.

In addition, magnesium can be lost in the cooking process. Water-softening agents remove magnesium (and calcium) from the water, and the boiling of vegetables will further destroy the mineral content. Also, oxalic acid (as in spinach) and phytic acid (as in cereal foods) tie up magnesium by forming salts that the body cannot absorb.

The symptoms of a magnesium deficiency are depression, irritability, muscle tremors and, occasionally, convulsive seizures accompanied by delirium. Adelle Davis in her book *Let's Get Well* states that a daily dose of 450 mg of magnesium, when used to treat epileptic patients, resulted in control of the seizures so that all drugs were discontinued. (Since this appears in her chapter on vitamin B-6, we suspect that magnesium plus adequate B-6 plus a better diet might have been the effective remedy.) Epileptic patients should certainly *not* have their anticonvulsant medications abruptly discontinued or replaced by magnesium oxide tablets. Continued seizures may result, with consequent brain damage. Dr. Pierre Muller, addressing the First International Symposium on Magnesium Deficit in Human Pathology in 1971, stated that data supports the belief that painful uterine contractions at the end of pregnancy are due to a deficiency of magnesium and suggested that a large number of premature interruptions of pregnancy may be related.

Fortunately, our kidneys are efficient in conserving magnesium. Therefore, unless one suffers from a kidney disease or loses an excessive amount of the mineral in sweat or feces, hypomagnesia is not likely to occur.

Where Can I Obtain Magnesium?

The National Academy of Sciences has set the RDA for magnesium at 350 mg for men, 300 for women, and 450 during pregnancy and lactation. Milk, nuts and whole grains are excellent sources of this essential mineral. Magnesium is found in green vegetables, particularly as part of the chorophyll molecule. Seafoods also contain appreciable amounts. The amount of magnesium obtained can be supplemented by taking dolomite, a naturally occurring mixture of calcium and magnesium.

References

Robinson, C. H. *Fundamentals of normal nutrition*. New York: Macmillan, 1973.

Schroeder, H. A., Nason. A. P. and Tipton, I. H. Essential metals in man: magnesium. *J. Chronic Dis.* vol. 21, 1969.

Seelig, M. S. Electrographic patterns of magnesium depletion appearing in alcoholic heart disease. *Annals of the New York Academy of Sciences* vol. 162: 2:906–917. 15 August 1969.

Wacker, E. C. and Vallee, B. L. Magnesium metabolism. *New Eng. J. of Med.* 259:9.

Magnesium Update 1978

A frequently successful treatment for eclampsia (convulsions and coma during and immediately following pregnancy) has been the administration of magnesium sulphate and sometimes B-6. The infants born of these mothers may experience acute depression or hypotonia (loss of body tone and firmness), and occasionally they are stillborn. Magnesium intoxication of infants can be avoided if the mother's urinary, serum and blood magnesium levels are carefully monitored.

Both magnesium hydroxide and magnesium trisilicate have been used as antacids and as a means of decreasing blood phosphate levels in renal patients on dialysis. Magnesium hydroxide toxicity results from phosphate depletion and is easily remedied by withdrawing the antacid and supplementing phosphate. Magnesium trisilicate should be avoided since there are significantly higher concentrations of silicon in the brains and hearts of patients who have died from Alzheimer's disease, arteriosclerosis and heart disease.

Magnesium (like zinc and manganese) in the U.S. diet has steadily decreased with the refining and processing of foods. The use of chelating agents in the preparation of frozen vegetables maintains greenness but results in a lowered magnesium content. Characteristics of deficiency are muscle tremors, convulsions, depression, poor memory, delirium and heart irregularities. Rats fed magnesium-deficient diets give birth to smaller rats with more congenital malformations, and they develop calcium deposits and other abnormalities within the heart cells. Magnesium deficiency in man is difficult to diagnose because of the ambiguity of the physiological symptoms—humans may maintain normal blood, serum and CSF magnesium levels even on a magnesium-deficient diet. As much as half the magnesium stored in bones may be released before a decrease in blood serum will occur. Magnesium is needed for mobilization of calcium from bone. Most body calcium and magnesium stores are in the skeletal system. A suggested test for deficiency is the intravenous injection of excess magnesium; a normal person excretes 90 percent of the magnesium, while a deficient person excretes less and absorbs more.

Magnesium deficiencies are often accompanied by hypocalcemia and hypokalemia (low potassium). There are many similarities between potassium and magnesium metabolism, although magnesium is much harder to displace from a cell than potassium. The concentration of potassium in cells is reduced by magnesium deficiency and does not return to normal until the magnesium deficiency has been corrected. Many dietary causes of magnesium deficiency are also causes of potassium deficiencies. Calcium supplements without adequate magnesium cannot prevent hypocalcemia.

Magnesium salts, the bicarbonate, carbonate, oxide, chloride and sulfate, all have been successful in treating deficiencies. (A calcium source is needed with prolonged doses of any of these salts.) Magnesium sulfate therapy has been particularly successful in treating convulsions of newborn babies.

The best dietary supplement is probably dolomite with pure bone meal, which provides adequate magnesium, calcium, phosphorus and other trace elements. Commercial bone meal should not be used as the exclusive source of calcium and magnesium, however, for such use can cause lead poisoning. Since many physicians do not consider the possibility of lead poisoning, it usually goes undiagnosed.

People living in regions with hard drinking water (plenty of magnesium and calcium carbonates) have a reduced risk of magnesium deficiency. These hard water areas also have a lessened incidence of heart disease and atherosclerosis.

References

Crosby, W. H. Lead-contaminated health food: association with lead poisoning and leukemia. *JAMA* 237:2627–2629, June 1977.

Davis, A. *Let's eat right to keep fit.* New York: Harcourt Brace Jovanovich, 1970, pp. 170–176.

Prasad, A. *Trace elements in human health and disease.* Vol. 2. New York: Academic Press, 1976, pp. 1–73.

Runeberg, L., et al. Hypomagnesemia due to renal disease of unknown etiology. *Am. J. of Med.* 59:873–880, 1975.

Turner, T. L., et al. Magnesium therapy in neonatal tetany. *The Lancet,* 5 February, 1977, pp. 283–284.

CHAPTER 9

Potassium

THOSE water pills that give relief from premenstrual tension and relieve water-logged tissues have the side-effect of producing potassium loss as well as salt (sodium) excretion. The daily intake of potassium may be marginal because some patients do not eat adequate amounts of vegetables and fruits which accumulate potash (potassium) from any well-nurtured soil. Symptoms of potassium deficiency are muscle weakness, fatigue, constipation and mental apathy. These symptoms will disappear when dietary changes provide sufficient potassium.

Studies show that the junk-food diet of high fat, refined sugars and oversalted food leads quickly to a state of potassium deficiency. In addition to those on water pills, patients on prednisone, ACTH, or digitalis require extra potassium. Patients with diabetes, high blood pressure or liver disease require a regular dietary supplement of potassium.

Foods particularly rich in potassium are green leafy vegetables, wheat germ, citrus juice, beans, lentils, nuts, dates, prunes and fruits of all kinds. With cooked vegetables, careful conservation of the pot liquor is necessary in order to minimize the water-soluble potassium loss. This pot liquor can be saved to make soups and broths or used immediately if the peas or beans are thickened with instant rice or instant rolled oats.

While these prepared foods have lost some potassium, they can nonetheless be restored with the vegetable water. If the vegetable water is used to cook rolled oats, then the potassium content should be even greater.

Pharmaceutical preparations of potassium chloride are Kaochlor liquid, Kay Ciel Elixir, K-Lor, K-Lyte-CL and Slow-K. Most of these are 10 percent flavored potassium chloride. Patients who take daily a full dose of a water pill (thiazide diuretic) may need three tablespoons of 10 percent potassium chloride each day. This dose can be reduced, however, by the careful selection of foods high in potassium. Potassium tablets irritate the stomach and cause pain. Enteric coated potassium can cause deep ulcers in the small intestine.

References

Kosman, M. E. Management of potassium problems during long-term diuretic therapy. *JAMA* 230:5, 4 November 1974.

Schwartz, A. B. and Swartz, C. D. Dosage of potassium chloride elixir to correct thiazide-induced hypokalemia. *JAMA* 230:5, 4 November 1974.

Potassium Update 1978

A recent newspaper headline read, "Physician drops dead while jogging." The physician was an orthomolecular psychiatrist who knew everything about vitamins but little about minerals. Optimal vitamin dosage requires optimal mineral intake which must be carefully tailored to provide the minerals lacking in our modern diet. These are potassium, magnesium, calcium, zinc, sulfur, selenium and sometimes manganese or molybdenum. Lack of one or more of these minerals apparently caused the doctor's heart to stop under the added demands of exercise. Many of our joggers get cramps in the calf muscles while jogging. This is a warning signal to drink a glass of orange or grapefruit juice before jogging, for the cramp in the calf may precede a cramp in the heart which can set off fatal fibrillation of the heart muscle. Karen Krautzcke, the champion tennis player, jogged as a form of relaxation after winning a tennis match in the Florida heat; tragically, potassium deficiency probably stopped her heart.

Some joggers are more fortunate. A shipping magnate, for example, had fainting spells after jogging and was hospitalized for a two-week period. He underwent the following perilous diagnostic tests: cardiac catheterization to visualize the heart vessels, carotid catheterization to visualize his brain and, of course, a brain wave study and brain scan. All proved negative, and so, after he adopted a better nutritional program, he started jogging again. This time he developed muscle cramps in the calf muscles—a clear warning of potassium deficiency. This symptom responded to a glass of grapefruit juice before his morning exercise.

Potassium is the major intracellular cation in the body and is man's most abundant mineral next to calcium and phosphorus. A 154-pound man has 9 ounces (300 grams) of potassium. Potassium works with sodium in the extracellular fluid to regulate blood pH, water balance, acidification of urine, nerve conduction and muscle contractions. Deficiency most commonly results from diuretic medication, ordinary diarrhea, vomiting and prolonged antibiotic use. Symptoms of deficiency include partial temporary paralysis or cramping of muscles, coma, cardiac arrythmia and infant colic. The medical terms for high and low potassium levels are hyper- and hypokalemia, respectively (kalemia deriving from the Latin word for potassium *kalium*). A deficiency can be detected by an ECG or a direct blood test. A normal diet should contain 2000 to 6000 mgs. Blood test values are given in milli-equivalents (normal range is 3.5 to 5.5 meq./liter).

Potassium Pills Pain the Stomach and Perforate the Intestine

The use of potassium pills can have serious side-effects. For example, potassium salts if encapsulated will disintegrate in the stomach and cause severe pain; the pain is quickly relieved, however, by an extra glass of water. On the other hand, potassium tablets that are enteric coated to bypass the stomach and liberate the potassium in the intestine may stay in one place too long and produce an ulcer of the intestine which perforates. Because of these potential side-effects, most potassium supplements are given in the form of effervescent tablets that must be mixed with water before swallowing. One can avoid problems with tablets altogether simply by eating fruits and vegetables which have bountiful amounts of potassium as well as extra trace elements (see Table 9.1). "K-lyte," the most frequently used potassium tablet, costs about 20 cents, which in the long run is more expensive than fruits and vegetables.

Water Pills (Diuretics) Reduce Sodium and Potassium

If thiazide diuretics (the usual water pills) are taken without large amounts of fruit, a potassium deficiency with paralysis can quickly result. Minor symptoms may be fatigue, muscle weakness or cramping. Anyone using diuretics should also avoid sodium chloride.

Compared to hypokalemia, hyperkalemia (excess potassium) is rare among Americans.

Sodium, Potassium and Heart Disease

Sodium and potassium help regulate the required equilibrium between the intra- and extracellular fluid. The body contains large potassium stores, 9 ounces (300 grams), but only 4 ounces (150 grams) of sodium.

TABLE 9.1

Foods rich in potassium

BEVERAGES mgm/100 ml or grams		FRUITS mgm/100 ml or grams	
Prune juice, canned	220	Peaches, raw, dried	900
Tomato juice	210	Banana	200
Orange juice, fresh	205		
Grapefruit juice, canned	200		
Grape juice, canned	160		
Pineapple juice, canned	160		
Apricot juice	155		
Milk, whole	140		
Milk, non-fat	110		

VEGETABLES mgm/100 ml or grams		FLOUR & WHEAT mgm/100 ml or grams	
Soybeans	400	Wheat germ	700
Red kidney beans	300	Soy flour	600
Carrots, diced, cooked	250	Whole wheat bread	200
Lentils	200		
Potato	200		

Much debated today is the question of what effects sodium and potassium have on blood pressure. Many tests have confirmed that sodium chloride contributes to high serum cholesterol and blood pressure. Small sustained changes in extracellular sodium concentration can have profound effects on arterial blood pressure. In the Virgin Islands, hypertension is endemic among natives who drink rain water collected on the hillside, a brackish water that contains sea spray from the ocean; blood pressure returns to normal levels when distilled water is used for drinking. Some individuals are less affected by high sodium chloride intake, probably because of their superior overall nutrition, specifically optimal intakes of potassium and calcium. In a recent study, longer life and lower blood pressure were the results of added potassium in the diet of cats on a high-salt diet. An increase of daily potassium intake in dogs, from a normal level of 30 meq/day to 200 meq/day, produced a 0.47 rise in plasma potassium with a 58 percent increase in sodium excretion. Clearly, then, potassium and sodium are antagonists. That potassium lowers the blood pressure has been confirmed only in a few human cases.

Salt hunger is not an inborn trait, but is culturally acquired. An African community, for instance, relies totally upon potassium chloride to salt food and prefers it even to the common salt (sodium chloride) Europeans introduced. Neither infants nor adults need sodium salted food; iodized potassium chloride and kelp should become the substitute. A particularly unhealthy practice is the salting of baby foods—a practice that is maintained simply to appeal to the mother's taste. Breast milk has a goodly amount of potassium: 55 mg per 100 ml (versus 15 mg per 100 ml of sodium).

Potassium and Exercise

An analysis of potassium levels in 116 trackmen demonstrated that 39 percent had resting hypokalemia. Vigorous exercise results in hyperkalemia, which is readily corrected in the two or three minutes following the strenuous exertion. During the subsequent post-recovery period, 60 percent of the runners suffered hypokalemia. A well-controlled study proved that in over four months of intensive training, potassium levels for trackmen dropped from 4.2 to 3.7, while the levels of untrained students decreased from 4.1 to 3.8 meq/liter after exercise.

The high protein diets eaten by athletes during training may contribute to potassium deficiency. On these diets nitrogen intake increases, with a resulting increase in sulfate and hydrochloride excretion. These acids are lost via the kidneys and urine with their full base equivalent of potassium. An unusual degree of muscular weakness and fatigue in the presence of a particularly good state of physical fitness indicates potassium problems. Athletes should include potassium-rich foods in their diet and take supplements when excessive sweating and fatigue result. "Gatorade," that highly advertised artificial thirst quencher, contains 5 calories, 1.38 grams carbohydrate, 16 mgm sodium, 3 mgm potassium and 2.1 mgm saccharin per fluid ounce; a salt tablet taken with a full glass of fruit juice is a better antidote to salt loss in hot weather.

Potassium and Magnesium

Magnesium and potassium deficiency often occur in alcoholics and the chronically ill. The potassium levels of a patient with deficient magnesium and potassium increased even when magnesium (which is essential for potassium retention) was the only supplement ingested, but in a similar case, supplements of potassium resulted in no correction of either deficiency. The best management of either deficiency should include dietary supplements of both potassium and magnesium.

Salt Substitutes

Most salt substitutes are based on high potassium chloride content. For example, Adolf's is 43 percent, Co-Salt 45 percent, Diasal 44 percent, Nu-Salt 40 percent and Salfree 55 percent potassium. Morton's "Lite Salt" is 26 percent potassium and 19.5 percent sodium, which is an improvement over an all-sodium salt. The other ingredients in "Lite Salt" are magnesium carbamate, 0.01 percent dextrose, potassium iodide and calcium polysilicate, none of which is harmful at the dosage used. Dried sea water ("sea salt") is 59 percent chloride, 33 percent sodium, 4 percent magnesium, 3 percent sulfur, 1 percent calcium, 1 percent potassium and small amounts of all elements of the earth. Not only is sea salt not a good source of potassium, but the sulfur it contains is in the form of the sulfate which provides sulfur to bacteria but not to man. While sea water and its nutrients were beneficial to cells when life began, sea salt for seasoning food is a poor bargain. Morton's salt substitute contains potassium chloride, fumaric acid (a natural body acid), tricalcium phosphate and mono-calcium phosphate. One whole teaspoon contains only 1 mgm of sodium and the flavoring effect is good. Most other salt substitutes are higher in sodium and contain mono-sodium or potassium glutamate (MSG), an undesirable substance for heart patients since glutamic acid is an amino acid that stimulates the heart rate.

Drs. Joseph A. Sopko and Richard M. Freeman report in the *Journal of the American Medical Association,* 15 August 1977, on the use of salt substitutes—a cheap and convenient source of potassium (potash). Morton's salt substitute costs about 3 cents for 4 grams, which gives 50 milli-equivalents. In contrast, the popular K-lyte effervescent tablets may cost almost 30 cents for the same dose of potassium. The K-lyte tablet, of course, contains artificial flavor and other additives that are not present in a simple salt substitute. The authors state that the salt substitutes are on the average ten to twelve times less expensive than the highly advertised potassium tablets, capsules and liquids. The use of a salt substitute will more closely approximate a timed-release dosage in that the user will perhaps salt (potash) the food three times a day, plus put potash on his egg during his morning break and on his ripe tomato during his afternoon break. Patients on the water pill may need 60 milli-equivalents or 5 grams per day (a level teaspoonful); Morton's salt substitute contains eighteen such level teaspoonfuls—all for 70 cents.

References

A.M.P. Bio-Research Institute. Sodium and potassium balance. 1(2):1–2, 1974.

Danilevicius, Z. Another form of iatrogenic hypokalemia. *JAMA* 236(23):2657, 1976.

Davis, A. *Let's eat right to keep fit.* New York: Signet, Signet Classics, Mentor and Plume Books, 1970.

Haddy, F. J. Potassium and blood vessels. *Life Sciences* 16:1489–1498, 1975.

Kosman, M. E. Management of potassium problems during longterm diuretic therapy. *JAMA* 230(5):743–748, 1974.

Macleod, S. M. The rational use of potassium supplements. *Post Graduate Medicine* 57(2):123–128, 1975.

Menelly, G. R. and Battaubee, H. D. Sodium and potassium. *Nutrition Reviews* 34(8): 225–235, 1976.

Newmark, S. R. and Dluhy, R. G. Hyperkalemia, hypokalemia. *Emergency Medicine* 1976, pp. 92–94.

Rose, K. D. Warning for millions: intense exercise can deplete potassium. *The Physician and Sports Medicine,* May 1975, pp. 67–70.

Sapir, D. G., et al. The role of potassium in the control of ammonium excretion during starvation. *Metabolism* 25(2):2210–2220, 1976.

Schwartz, A. B. Therapy of hypokalemia. *Clinical Pharmacology* 13(4):148–149, 1976.

Whang, R. and Aikawa, J. K. Magnesium deficiency and refractoriness to potassium repletion. *J. Chron. Dis.* 30:65–68, 1977.

Winsor, T. Electrolyte abnormalities and the electrocardiogram. *JAMA* 203:4–6, 1968.

Young, D. B., et al. The natriuretic and hypotensive effects of potassium, Supp. II. *Circ. Res.* 38(6):84–89, 1976.

CHAPTER 10

Molybdenum

ONE of the more difficult names to spell, molybdenum is an essential trace element, important to human life. It is a silvery-gray metal that looks something like lead, is used in ferro-alloys in small proportions (molybdenum steel hack saws) and is mined, almost exclusively, in one large deposit in Colorado.

Life Would Not Be Possible Without Molybdenum

In the nitrogen-fixation process, molybdenum is an essential catalyst, since bacteria-fixing atmospheric nitrogens require its chemical attributes to begin protein synthesis. Where molybdenum is lacking in the soil, the land is barren. When molybdenum-containing fertilizers are added to lawns, this will encourage clover, with its nitrogen-fixing root nodules, to thrive. (If you want an all-clover lawn, then use molybdenum plus some vanadium!)

Molybdenum is essential to all mammals; it is in all of our tissues. Three important enzymes need molybdenum. Deficiencies are a distinct possibility in man, since our main source of caloric energy—fats and carbohydrates—have molybdenum only in whole grains or wheat germ. We process these grains, of course. Our white flour has lost its molybdenum to the bran (which is fed to chickens and cattle). Our refined sugar has lost its molybdenum to molasses. Only a judicious choice of protein foods and vegetables will ensure adequate amounts of the trace metal in the remaining caloric intake.

Like fluorine, molybdenum appears to prevent dental caries. When U.S. Navy recruits from Ohio were found to be surprisingly free of dental cavities, this was traced to the molybdenum in foods which came from the Ohio soil.

Molybdenum may also be responsible for lack of esophageal cancer in many parts of the world. In the Transkei region of South Africa, where cancer of the esophagus is increasing at an epidemic rate, researchers have found that indigenous vegetation is highly deficient in molybdenum. In the United States, areas deficient in molybdenum also had high rates of cancer of the esophagus. A third condition which might be the upshot of molybdenum deficiency is sexual impotency in older males.

Molybdenum overload or poisoning in humans is very unusual, even when the metal is inhaled as industrial fumes. However, sheep and cattle grazing on molybdenum-rich pasture may develop a copper deficiency. This is evidenced, in black sheep, by lack of pigment in their wool. With alternation of high molybdenum or high copper in the black sheep's diet, one can produce wool which is banded black and white. This demonstrates the dependency of copper metabolism on molybdenum intake, although the exact role of each mineral is an enigma. Conversely, a copper overload may be corrected by administering molybdenum. (Actually, the interaction is tripartite, involving sulfur as well.)

Molybdenum is obtainable in a number of foods. It also can be purchased as drops which can be added to milk or water. A good commercial source of molybdenum is Mol-Iron, which contains both molybdenum and iron.

TABLE 10.1

Food sources of molybdenum

Mcg%

Grain		Meal	
Buckwheat	485	Buckwheat	8
Oats	114	Corn	9
Corn	50	Wheat	50
Cornflakes	8	Soybean	182
Barley	138		
Rice	47	**Fruits**	
Wheat	60	Apple	Trace
Wheat germ	200	Apricot	14
Soybean	—	Banana	3
		Cantaloupe	16
Bread		Plums	6
Whole wheat	30	Raisins	11
White	21	Strawberry	9
Rye	50		
		Vegetables	
Prepared foods		Lima beans	400
		Canned beans	350
Noodles	45	Lentils	120
Macaroni	51	Green beans	66
Molasses	18	Yams	59
		Potato	25
Nuts		Carrots	8
		Celery	2
Coconut	25	Lettuce	2
Sunflower seeds	103	Spinach	26
		Endive	4
Miscellaneous		Watercress	10
		Zucchini	12
Butter	10	Eggplant	—
Eggs	50	Green peppers	—
Milk	3	Tomato	—
Milk powder	14	Onions	—
Honey	—		
Cheese	5	**Meats**	
Cocoa	50	Chicken	40
Coffee	—	Hearts	75
Tea	8	Liver	200
Wine	5	Kidney	75
Beer	6	Fish	4
Scotch whisky	17	Shellfish	20

Some mineral waters in Switzerland have high levels of molybdenum (Eglisau—25 to 52 mcg/1 and Bex—26.5 mcg/1). Drinking water only has traces of molybdenum except in the S-charl region of Switzerland (29.0 mcg/1).

Source: D. Schlettwein-Gsell and S. Mommsen-Straub. Ubersichtsartikel spurenelemente in Lebensmitteln X. Molybdan. *International Journal for Vitamin and Nutrition Research 43:*110, 1973.

References

Brody, J. E. Dietary factors linked to cancer of digestive tract. *The New York Times* p. 24, 29 September 1972.

Schroeder, H. A., Balassa, J. J. and Tipton, I. H. Essential trace metals in man: molybdenum. *J. Chron. Dis.* 23:481, 1970.

Molybdenum Update 1978

There is increasing evidence that molybdenum deficiency can be a causative factor in human disease. xanthine oxidase is the main body enzyme which requires molybdenum for action. However, in man the level of xanthine, uric acid, is lowered only at high intakes of molybdenum (10 to 15 mg/d). In a study of two populations, high molybdenum/low copper was associated with decreased dental caries when fluoride intake was stable in both groups. The population with a low incidence of caries also had high vanadium levels. Under usual conditions man's minimum requirement of molybdenum is small, perhaps as little as 120 ug/day.

Populations on high molybdenum foods (varieties of sorghum) might show clinical symptoms resulting from deficiences of copper. Conversely, low molybdenum diets might be expected to show clinical symptoms of copper toxicity.

High tungsten will result in a molybdenum type of deficiency (tungsten can replace molybdenum in certain important enzymes in mammals). Tungsten substitution for molybdenum results in inactive or weak biologically active enzymes. Tungsten poisoning may result in clinical symptoms of high copper because the molybdenum would be inactivated.

It has been found that dietary molybdenum lowers plasma phosphorus excretion in sheep and increases phosphorus excretion in cattle, most of the phosphorus being excreted in the feces. The antagonism of phosphorus and molybdenum in man has not yet been determined.

The Brain Bio Center continues to use the prescription drug Mol-iron as a source of molybdenum in patients. Cancer of the esophagus and stomach may be prevented by molybdenum. The only side-effect of a large molybdenum dosage is a tightness and increased tone of the large muscles of the body such as the back, hips and thighs. Inasmuch as excess molybdenum decreases growth in all species studied, molybdenum levels should particularly be investigated in teen-agers with run-away bone growth at the expense of their physical and psychic health.

References

Dental caries prevalence and trace elements other than fluoride. *Nutrition Reviews* 32:120–122, 1974.

Deosthale, Y. G. and Gopalen, C. The effect of molybdenum levels in sorghum (Sorghum vulgare Pers) on uric acid and copper excretion in man. *Br. J. Nutr.* 31:351–355, 1974.

Ljungdahl, L. G. Tungsten: a biologically active metal. *TIBS*, March 1976, pp. 63–64.

Pitt, M. A. Molybdenum toxicity: interactions between copper, molybdenum and sulphate. *Agents and Actions* 6:758–769, 1976.

Schroeder, H. A.; Balassa, J. J. and Tipton, I. H. Essential trace metals in man: molybdenum. *J. Chron. Dis.* 23:481–499, 1970.

CHAPTER 11

Vanadium: Little-known Element

ONE of our earliest ancestors was the *Amphioxas*, a cross between a fish and a worm, a link between vertebrates and invertebrates. This first chordate fish had a spinal cord with a slight bulge on the end which, over the millenia, developed into the human brain. The *Amphioxas* was fortunate in choosing iron as the chief transporter of oxygen in its blood, for, through some evolutionary quirk, a very close relative of the *Amphioxas* was forced to use vanadium for this purpose. Vanadium, more limited in availability than iron, produced an evolutionary regression; the *Amphioxas* became us, while its close relative became the common sea squirt. Instead of red blood cells full of iron, the squirt has green blood cells full of vanadium. And while the larvae of the squirt still have ganglionic bulges on their spinal cords, the mature squirts do not—hence they are brainless.

One may appreciate the presence of iron in one's hemoglobin and pity the poor sea squirt, who somewhere along the line was cut off from a supply of iron and lost his chance to have a brain. But one need not fear vanadium. (Ingesting vanadium will not make your blood green, nor will it shrink your brain and turn you into a sea squirt!) Vanadium is an element that is present throughout the human body. At maximum possible intake from trace amounts in dietary sources and air pollution, vanadium has no known toxicity.

Nutritional studies from four laboratories have shown beyond a doubt that vanadium is an essential trace element for both the rat and the chicken. One study conducted by Hopkins and Mohr in 1970 demonstrated that a vanadium-deficient diet produced a significant loss of feather growth in young chickens. He also showed that a vanadium deficiency decreases the reproduction rate in rats and increases mortality in their offspring. Other independent studies have shown that vanadium is essential to the growth of rats. Vanadium can be assumed to be essential to humans as well, because it is rapidly used by the body and excreted in the urine and it is found in most tissues. All other elements with these same properties, such as zinc, have been found essential. The dietary need for animals is 0.2 ppm. Many animal diets do not reach this level.

Sources of Vanadium

Vanadium is highly concentrated in fats and vegetable oils. At high levels, it helps to lower serum cholesterol, particularly in people of middle age. Vanadium shares with chromium and zinc this cholesterol-lowering ability. Like molybdenum, it is needed by the nitrogen-fixing bacteria of the soil. Another source of vanadium is the burning of coal and certain types of crude oil; there need not be concern for this particular air pollutant. Although vanadium accumulates in the lungs with age, it has little toxicity and apparently no adverse effect on longevity.

Nutrients and Evolution

The probable need for vanadium in human nutrition is one more reason to rise to the challenge of maintaining natural, nutrient-rich diets. Little-known elements such as vanadium are certainly not restored to processed foods after they have been stripped away in the food factory, and yet they occur readily in nature and in unprocessed foods.

Trace elements are the nutrients man evolved on, abundant in our diets and those of our ancestors for all but the last twenty of the many millions of years it took life to evolve. In these past twenty years, food processing and high-yield farming techniques have caused depletion in the amounts of these nutrients found in our foods.

And who knows? Long after the human race has disappeared from earth, perhaps sea squirts will evolve a new race of green-blooded, vanadium-rich, intelligent creatures who put too much vanadium back in their processed foods after stripping away all the iron!

References

A new essential trace element—vanadium. *Medical News, JAMA* 222:3:255–256, 16, October 1972.

Hopkins, L. L. and Mohr, H. E. Vanadium as an essential nutrient. *Fed. Proc.* 33:1773, 1973.

Schroeder, H. A. *The trace elements and man.* Old Greenwich, Connecticut: Devin–Adair, 1973.

Schwarz, K. and Milne, D. B. Growth effects of vanadium in the rat. *Science* 174:426–428, 22 October 1971.

Vanadium Update 1978

Nutritional studies on vanadium have demonstrated that high vanadium diets lower plasma phospholipid levels in animals and inhibit cholesterol synthesis in human subjects younger than middle age. Vanadium-deficient diets result in increased triglyceride levels in chickens. The means by which vanadium exerts an effect on lipid metabolism is unknown.

The value of vanadium in preventing dental caries has not been clearly established. Although radioactive vanadium concentrates in the bones and teeth of rats, administration of vanadium through drinking water has not resulted in any decrease in animal dental caries. (Untampered water or mineral water supplies have varied vanadium concentrations according to geographical area.)

Other experiments involving chickens and rats have demonstrated chromium and possible sulfur antagonism by vanadium.

Foods with appreciable levels of vanadium are black pepper, soybean oil, corn oil, olive oil, olives and gelatine. The focus of future research is on the value and need of vanadium in human nutrition.

References

Myron, D. R., et al. Vanadium content of selected foods as determined by flameless atomic absorption spectroscopy. *J. of Agric. Food Chem.* 25(2):297–299, 1977.

Underwood, E. J. *Trace elements in human and animal nutrition.* 4th ed. New York: Academic Press, 1977.

CHAPTER 12

Chromium

Chromium-Glucose Tolerance Factor Essential for Burning Blood Sugar

A CERTAIN desert rodent, the sand rat, develops sugar diabetes when raised on laboratory food. When the sand rat is returned to the desert, its diabetic condition disappears. What is the key nutrient missing from rat food which the rat finds in its natural forage? Extensive laboratory analyses indicate that it is *chromium*. Chromium bound in an organic form in the glucose tolerance factor (GTF) potentiates the effect of insulin on glucose intake and so suppresses the latent diabetes of the sand rat. The salt-bush which is hoarded by the rat in its burrows contains enough GTF to prevent diabetes.

Other trace elements contained in the salt-bush and known to have a hypoglycemic effect are manganese, zinc, calcium, potassium and sodium. Manganese, zinc and chromium are the most effective. Chromium is known to be essential to the effectiveness of the insulin hormone.

Dr. Walter Mertz of the Human Nutrition Laboratory in Beltsville, Maryland has spent the last fifteen years studying chromium and its availability to human life. Dr. Mertz has found that with glucose, as in the glucose tolerance test (GTTest), the chromium level of the blood rises with the glucose (blood sugar) level. With this glucose load, significant amounts of chromium are excreted in the urine and lost to the body. The GTTest is stressful, while sugars slowly released from fruits and vegetables would not dissipate the GTF and might even have enough GTF to take care of the contained starches and sugars.

Chromium Deficiency

In Western countries the body content of chromium decreases with age, while in Eastern countries where natural foods are eaten the chromium content is maintained. Many women in Western countries are so deficient in chromium that the white blood cell chromium level may decrease by 50 percent with each pregnancy, resulting first in complete alcohol intolerance and later in glucose intolerance (adult-type diabetes). The two best sources of chromium are brewer's yeast and sugar beet molasses. Because this molasses is less sweet than cane molasses, it is seldom marketed, and that leaves brewer's yeast as the best available source.

Glucose Tolerance Factor

Humans, like rats, need this glucose tolerance factor (GTF). GTF is an organic chromium compound whose exact chemical structure is now being determined. Trivalent chromium is known to be the center of the molecule which also contains two niacin molecules (vitamin B-3) and three amino acids. These amino acids are now known to be glutamic acid and glycine and cysteine. The scientists at Beltsville have tried to put this jigsaw puzzle together. Now that they have crystallized the GTF from commercial brewer's yeast they can subject the crystals to X-ray analysis and so disclose the exact configuration of the two niacins, three amino acids and the trivalent chromium. GTF works with the hormone insulin to maintain the delicate balance between hypoglycemic (low blood sugar) and hyperglycemic (high blood sugar) conditions. Glucose is required for every cellular function. It supplies the energy that is burned every time a muscle contracts or a nerve impulse is transmitted.

The pure GTF is completely nontoxic when given by mouth or even intravenously to the mouse and rat. Yet it is now undergoing chronic toxicity studies to determine whether that which has been separated from brewer's yeast is toxic when administered over a long period of time! That's silly, of course, but that's the way the food and drug laws are written. Because of having to work within these legal restrictions, the pure GTF is not yet available for use in man. In the meantime we must all take six brewer's yeast tablets morning and night if we wish to make sure we get enough of this new vitamin which contains chromium.

A similar vitamin, B-12, contains cobalt rather than chromium. B-12 is the only vitamin which must be given by injection because absorption from the intestines is so poor. GTF is well absorbed by mouth both in man and in animals, so injection will not be necessary. The human dose of pure GTF is now estimated to be 2 to 6 mg per day by mouth. GTF is not entirely new since brewer's yeast and soluble chromium salts have been used to lower the insulin requirement of unstable diabetic children and also to get older patients off insulin and oral insulin substitutes.

GTF is then a trivalent chromium in an organic chemical complex which cannot be easily synthesized in the body but may be synthesized by the normal bacteria of the intestine when enough chromium is contained in the diet. Older people in Western nations are depleted of their GTF and need a good dietary source. Eventually $Cr+++$ will be shifted from rare-trace-metal-nutrient status to full-fledged-vitamin status since adequate synthesis in the human body is questionable.

If you think the GTtest is stressful, imagine what happens to the GTF when glucose 5 percent or 10 percent is given intravenously to nourish the patient in the postoperative period. Pacarek and his colleagues have found that the blood chromium drops precipitously when 60 gm of glucose is given intravenously—for example, 600 ml of 10 percent glucose. If the postoperative patient also has a virus infection, the blood chromium may drop to one-third (from 1.49 to 0.45 ppb). If the patient is then given intravenous glucose, the end results might be disastrous. Our hypoglycemic patients avoid hospitals and put off needed elective operations in justified fear of the intravenous glucose which may be given like the daily bath whether the patient needs it or not!

With Dr. Mertz's discovery we should have the GTF available in the 5 to 10 percent glucose, perhaps with a trace-element nutrient solution containing at least zinc, calcium, magnesium and manganese. The evidence for the need for each of these with GTF in glucose metabolism is scientifically solid—so why wait? Because of the food and drug laws, we must wait until scientific intravenous nutrition is slowly justified—at great expense.

Brewer's Yeast for GTF

Simple measurements of the chromium content of food can be misleading because chromium occurs in several forms with the range of oral absorption between 1 percent and 10 percent. Inorganic chromium is only 1 percent absorbable or less. Eggs have a high chromium concentration, but little of their chromium content is in the organic form biologically available as GTF. Chromium-containing foods with biologically active chromium are brewer's yeast, black pepper, liver, beef, whole-wheat bread, beets, beet sugar molasses, mushrooms and beer. Among these, far and away the highest in chromium content is brewer's yeast. For the patient suspected of impaired glucose tolerance, brewer's yeast tablets are an indispensable supplement in the diet.

Questions to Be Answered

Since the GTF contains two molecules of niacin and

since some schizophrenics respond to extra niacin and many schizophrenics have impaired glucose tolerance, we must work harder to correlate one or more of the schizophrenias with deficiency of niacin or of the GTF or both. Do large doses of niacin make trivial dietary amounts of chromium more effective? Will the GTF be effective in the hypoglycemias or only in diabetes? Is any type of mental disorder produced by deficiency in the GTF? All of these questions and more must be answered.

We know that certain vegetables will form the GTF when the soil is supplemented with the chromium ion. Perhaps further supplementation with niacin and chromium might allow more of the GTF to be formed. At least, the riddle is almost solved, and we look forward to the time when pure GTF will be available for use in schizophrenic and hypoglycemic patients and in diabetics.

References

Jennings, J. Diet, hormones and diabetes. *Prevention* p. 83, December 1971.

Hambidge, K. M. Chromium nutrition in man. *Amer. J. Clin. Nutr.* 27:505 May 1974.

Mertz, W. Chromium occurrence and function in biological systems. *Phys. Rev.* 49:163, April 1969.

Mertz et al. *Fed. Proc.* 33:659, 1974.

Pecarek, R. S. et al. *Anal. Biochemistry* 59:283, 1974.

——*Fed. Proc.* 33:660, 1974.

——Relationship between serum chromium concentrations and glucose utilization in normal and infected subjects. *Diabetes* 24:350, 1975.

Schroeder, H. A. et al. Chromium deficiency as a factor in atherosclerosis. *J. Chron. Dis.* 23:123, 1970.

Chromium Update 1978

Chromium has been found to be essential to both the growth and longevity of laboratory animals. Studies done on mice and rats showed that male mice and rats receiving 2 or 5 ppm chromium in their drinking water grew significantly better than their controls. The median age of the male mice and rats was 99 and 91 days longer, respectively, than the control animals. No such effect was detected for females.

Another site of chromium action is the eye. Rats ingesting low chromium and protein diets developed an opaque cornea and congestion of the iridial vessels.

In man, chromium deficiency may be a factor in arteriosclerosis and hypertension (Table 12.1).

In addition to disturbing glucose and lipid (cholesterol) metabolism, it inhibits protein synthesis. The amino acids most affected by chromium deficiency are alpha-aminoisobutyric acid, glycine, serine and methionine.

While it is difficult to analyze chromium nutrition in human beings, hair analysis has provided a useful comparison of chromium nutritional status since changes in chromium concentration seem to parallel those in other tissues (Table 12.2). Evaluation of urine excretion can also indicate deficiencies. Chromium-deficient patients do not have the customary increase in urinary chromium excretion following oral glucose.

TABLE 12.1

Average postmortem liver chromium mg/gm of 92 patients

Controls	12.7
Hypertension	10.2
Arteriosclerosis	9.6
Diabetes	8.6

TABLE 12.2

Average hair chromium ppb (parts per billion)

Subject	Average Age	Sex	Chromium
Nulliparous (No Children)	29.7	F	309
Parous (After Children)	32.4	F	117
Controls	43	97% F	241
Diabetics	43	97% F	94
Normal newborns	0	M & F	910
Normal size premature newborns	30-36 weeks	M & F	325
Small size premature newborns	30-36 weeks	M & F	154
Infants	7 months	M & F	880
Infants	10-12 months	M & F	650
Infants	12-24 months	M & F	540
Infants	24-36 months	M & F	400

Although inorganic chromium compounds ($CrCl_3$) are poorly absorbed (1 to 3 percent), they are very effective in treating kwashiorkor children and marasmic [progressive emaciation] infants. In normal patients there is usually a three-week delay before the inorganic chromates have effect, though in one case the effect of $CrCl_3$ was immediate.

It has been estimated that 10 to 25 percent of the GTF in brewer's yeast is absorbed. Since structural analysis of GTF has not yet been completed, it has not been marketed. Long-term studies, however, have revealed a number of its properties and actions. For example, GTF is apparently non-toxic; it most resembles a hormone; and it is released into the blood in response to insulin and is then transported to the periphery of the insulin target tissue where it becomes involved in sugar utilization.

The availability of circulatory chromium appears to decrease during any acute infection. The body's use of chromium to inhibit antibody responses could explain the altered glucose tolerance curve characteristic of infections.

References

Benjanuvatra, N. K.; Bennin, M., et al. Hair chromium concentration of Thai subjects, with and without diabetes mellitus. *Nut. Reports International* 12(5):325–330, 1975.

Figoni, R. A. and Treagan, L. Inhibitory effect of nickel and chromium upon antibody response of rats to immunization with T–1 phage. *Research Communication in Chemical Pathology and Pharmacology* 11(2):335–338, 1975.

Hambidge, K. M. Chromium nutrition in man. *Am. J. of Clin. Nut.* 27:505–514, 1974.

Jeejeebhoy, K. N., et al. Chromium deficiency, glucose intolerance, and neuropathy reversed by chromium supplementation in a patient receiving long-term total parenteral nutrition. *Am. J. of Clin. Nut.* 30:531–538, 1977.

Mahalko, J. R. and Bennion, M. The effect of parity and time between pregnancies on maternal hair chromium concentration. *Am. J. of Clin. Nut.* 29:1069–1072, 1976.

Mertz, W. Effects and metabolism of glucose tolerance factor. *Nutrition Reviews* 33(5):129–135, 1975.

Morgan, J. M. Hepatic chromium content in diabetic subjects. *Metabolism* 21:313–316, 1972.

Pecarek, R. S., et al. Relationship between serum chromium concentrations and glucose utilization in normal and infected subjects. *Diabetes* 24(4):350–353, 1975.

Underwood, E. J. *Trace elements in human and animal nutrition*, 4th ed. New York: Academic Press, 1977, Ch. 10, pp. 258–269.

CHAPTER 13

Tin

TIN was discovered to be an essential life element during the 1960s; however, the nature of its specific functions is debatable. Because of its widespread use in industry, tin has a high potential for atmospheric pollution. Higher levels are therefore found in the lungs than in any other tissues. More lung tin is found in people in highly industrialized areas of the country than in other areas.

Apparently only a mildly poisonous effect results from the inhalation or ingestion of tin salts. Stannous chloride is an example of a tin salt which is found frequently as a chemical preservative. Stannous fluoride is present in some toothpastes. The average daily consumption by man, as indicated by food analysis on a collection of samples, is approximately 2 mg. Attempts to determine normal tissue and body tin content have been hindered by two problems: the destruction of the structure of the chemical complexes of tin during the process of ashing the sample, and lack of adequate research into the nature of tin complexes or molecules in biological samples.

Diets containing high levels of tin can frequently cause anemia unless sufficient amounts of iron are given. Experiments have shown that in rats, 0.3 percent tin in the diet caused growth depression and lowered the amount of hemoglobin synthesized. In this study, some histological changes occurred in the liver. These effects were diminished by administration of copper and iron. Therefore, one might conclude that tin does not work in the body system in isolation but is affected by other trace metals, particularly iron and copper.

Since tinplate is widely used in the canning of foods, continued research efforts should be made to determine whether tin is entirely innocuous. One report has stated that asparagus spears had a different taste when canned in glass jars. The preferable taste was restored when traces of tin were added to asparagus in glass jars.

References

Dekker, M. *Newer trace elements in nutrition.* New York: Mertz and Cornatzer, 1947.

Hiles, R. Absorption, distribution and excretion of inorganic tin in rats. *Toxicity and Applied Pharmacology* 27:366–379, 1974.

Trager, J. *The bellybook.* New York: Grossman, 1972.

Tin Update 1978

When 1 to 2 ppm of the tin salt stannic sulfate was added to the drinking water of rats, an increase of nearly 60 percent in growth rate resulted. Tin may therefore be an essential nutrient for the growth of rats.

Foods in tin-plated sheet metal cans that have no internal coating have tin levels ranging from 9 to 700 ppm. Apparently, such cans are not toxic, for the last reported case of tin poisoning was in 1949. At any rate, the toxic effects of tin are not usually serious because absorption is slow and retention is very poor.

Disorders related to tin deficiency in man have not been reported, and the biological chemistry of the element remains an enigma. The absence of recent nutritional research on tin prevents any further advice to the consumer.

References

Hiles, R. A. Absorption, distribution and excretion of inorganic tin in rats. *Toxicology and Applied Pharmacology* 27:366–379, 1974.

Underwood, E. J. *Trace elements in human and animal nutrition.* New York: Academic Press, 1977, Ch. 19.

CHAPTER 14

Cobalt

COBALT is essential for life as a vital part of the vitamin B-12 molecule. No other function of cobalt in animal or man is known. Dr. Henry A. Schroeder believes that humans do not need to worry about cobalt deficiency because humans require very little of this trace metal and we receive adequate supplies from animal sources. Thus, we need only worry about B-12 deficiency in strict vegetarians and older people. No evidence of cobalt insufficiency has been observed in humans, even in cases where there was not enough cobalt in the soil to keep plant-eating sheep and cattle healthy.

Beginning in 1935, mysterious wasting diseases afflicted cattle and sheep in areas of Australia and New Zealand. After a long and exhaustive investigation, a chain of nutritional insufficiencies was traced. In 1948, vitamin B-12 was discovered to contain cobalt. The soil in the areas of affliction was found to be deficient in cobalt. Local plants, therefore, were deficient in that mineral and the plants failed to supply the animals with amounts of cobalt needed for sufficient B-12 production.

Cobalt Excess

In 1966, another strange new disease, which culminated in heart failure, struck heavy beer drinkers in Quebec City, Canada; Leuven, Belgium; Omaha, Nebraska; and Minneapolis, Minnesota. Various physicians and researchers voiced opinions as to the cause. Some attributed this disease of the heart muscle to an excess of cobalt. Others thought other dietary factors were involved and that cobalt was not solely responsible, and Dr. C. A. Alexander noted that many of the victims had inadequate diets, especially low in protein. These tragic victims were consuming between six and thirty bottles of beer per day, and the *Annals of Internal Medicine* reported that 1.2 ppm of cobalt were found in the Canadian beer. The film left on the glassware by synthetic detergents kills the foamy "head" of beer. Therefore, cobalt was added to beer to preserve the foamy head and keep the product aesthetically pleasing.

As "beer drinkers' cardiomyopathy" illustrates, too much cobalt can be toxic. Administering too much cobalt has caused polycythemia (too many red blood cells) in rats, mice, guinea pigs, ducks, chickens, pigs, dogs and humans.

It is interesting that G. S. Wiburg et al. have found that a high-quality protein diet gave considerable protection against the toxicity of cobalt. Nutrition must continue to be a complete picture, not just a couple of spotlighted items.

References

Alexander, C. A. Cobalt-beer cardiomyopathy. *Amer. J. Med.* October 1972.

Cobalt and the heart, *Annals of Int. Med.* 70:2, February 1969.

Wiburg, G. S. et al. Factors affecting the cardiotoxic potential of cobalt. *Clinical Toxicology* 2(3):257–271, September 1969.

Cobalt Update 1978

Cobalt chloride has been successful in stimulating red blood cell production in anemia resulting from inflamed kidneys or infection. Cobalt-iron compounds have also been helpful in treating iron-deficiency anemia in children and pregnant women. The large doses (20 to 30 mg) of cobalt chloride needed to alleviate this anemia often proves toxic, however. Cobalt salts have limited, if any, value in human nutrition.

References

Underwood, E. J. *Trace elements in human and animal nutrition*. New York: Academic Press, Inc., 1977, Ch. 5.

CHAPTER 15

Fluoride

ELEMENTAL fluorine is a highly reactive, greenish-yellow gas and therefore never occurs alone in nature; the fluoride ion, however, is common and occurs in minerals bonded to metals to make binary fluoride salts. The wide distribution of these salts in the ocean and soil is responsible for the presence of fluoride in all body tissues. Fluoride has never been proven essential to life, but it is important in human nutrition to help maintain normal bone and tooth structure and resistance of teeth to decay. Fluoride has been administered alone to curb osteoporosis (a decrease in bone density) and to stop the loss of hearing associated with otosclerosis. Its most extensive and widely publicized use has been as an additive to public drinking water.

The Fluoridation Debate

Fluoridation may be traced back to Colorado Springs and the year 1916. There, a dentist named Frederick S. McKay noticed mottled teeth, but few cavities, in his patients. The city's water supply was analyzed and found to contain 2 ppm of fluoride as soluble salts. (Optimal for good tooth structure is 1 ppm.) Subsequent surveys throughout the world revealed a definite inverse relationship between incidence of dental caries and fluoride concentration in drinking waters. Excessive fluoride intake, however, was found to cause mottled teeth. This condition is characterized by chalky white splotches over the surface of the teeth combined with intermittent yellow-brown staining. In severe cases, there is pitting of the enamel which causes the teeth to appear corroded.

The incidence of dental caries and the incidence of mottling as functions of fluorine concentration were carefully plotted on a logarithmic scale. The two lines crossed at 1 ppm, which became the standard value for "eufluorosis." This condition occurs when there is optimum protection against dental caries with a minimum of mottling. Now hundreds of municipalities have fluoridated their water supplies to maintain fluoride levels of 0.8 to 1.2 ppm. For areas of higher mean temperature (more sweating and therefore more drinking) less fluoride is needed. Fluoridation has produced average reductions of 40 to 70 percent in the incidence of dental caries in children born after the treatment started.

Still, hundreds of communities refrain from adding fluoride to their water. Opponents of fluoridation maintain that we already receive enough fluoride from other sources. Tea, for example, is rich in fluorine, and many industries emit fluorine fumes in processing minerals. Opponents cite cases where cows have grazed on fluoride-rich pasture and have become exceedingly crippled. They also cite cases where tooth mottling occurs. Tooth decay, they maintain, is a disease of civilization caused by our excessive intake of sweets and carbohydrates, and fluoridation is only a ploy to keep soft-drink and candy industries in business. Those who sweat excessively and drink only soft drinks are apt to be fluoride-treatment failures.

On the other hand, statistics show that the benefits of fluoridation far outweigh their costs; fluorosis (fluoride poisoning), mottling and other ill effects have been minimal as long as fluoride levels are monitored, supervised and maintained in the neighborhood of 1 ppm. Anthropologists have demonstrated that tooth decay has occurred in all agricultural people throughout history, whether they had access to sweets and junk foods or not. And finally, the foremost trace elements experts universally and independently concur that fluoridation of water supplies is generally beneficial. These scientists are Navia of Alabama, Schroeder of Vermont, Mertz of Maryland and Underwood of Australia.

Fluoride in toothpaste is most effective before it is diluted by saliva, when it comes directly in contact with teeth and can inhibit bacterial growth. Direct contact with the teeth is also the means by which fluoridated waters reduce caries. Good food sources of fluoride include fish, cheese, and meat as well as tea.

References

Shupe, J. L., Olson, A. E., Sharma, R. P. Fluoride toxicity in domestic and wild animals. *Clinical Toxicology* 5:195, 1972.

Sodium fluoride halts otosclerosis hearing loss. *JAMA* 224:1482, 11 June 1973.

Underwood, E. J. *Trace elements in human and animal nutrition.* New York: Academic Press, 1971.

Fluoride Update 1978

The value of fluoride in human nutrition is controversial, and the literature on it is marked by contradiction. For every positive assertion as to its value in our diet there is a corresponding denial; hence, the health profession is divided into those who claim fluoridation of the water supply is poison and those who call it a panacea. The debate focuses on the role of fluoride in bone development and maintenance, and in dental health. Other topics that are disputed, though less studied, are the role of fluoride in cancer, heart disease, congenital malformations and fluoride intoxication.

Ingested fluoride is built into the tooth and bone structure. In experimenting on mice, Schroeder has reported that a fluoride supplement of 10 ppm fluorine in drinking water increased body weight and longevity. Highly purified diets supplemented with 1, 2.5 and 7.5

ppm fluoride resulted in a 30 percent increase in rat growth. In other experiments, fluorine was eliminated from the diet without effecting any change in normal skeletal growth.

Bone Strength

The value of fluoride in treating various forms of osteoporosis (reduced density of bone mass) has not yet been conclusively demonstrated. Some workers given fluoride reported beneficial effects on back pains, bone density and calcium balance, while others reported adverse reactions with fluoride therapy or failed to show an improved calcium balance. For many patients in whom fluoride was believed to halt osteoporosis, the diet included extra phosphate, vitamin D and/or calcium.

A frequent observation is that fluoride prevents hearing loss in elderly people with otosclerosis (new formations of spongy tissue that results in progressive deafness). The inhibiting action is thought to be a result of accumulated fluorine in small bones of the ear. Another study, however, cites this very same storage capacity of bones as an eventual cause of otosclerosis. The only point of general agreement is that the skeleton has the capacity to immobilize safely and to retain small amounts of fluoride, acting as a buffer against systemic effects. The storage capacity decreases with age and increases with skeletal growth.

Dental Caries

Many studies have examined the incidence of dental caries in populations with non-fluoridated versus fluoridated water or with high fluorine diets versus low fluorine diets. These studies have confirmed a lower rate of caries formation and the possibility of long-lasting benefit. Most of these studies have ignored the fact that high fluorine diets result in an initial delay wherein fluoride affects the tooth germ, causing a delay in dentition. Schatz has shown that dental caries develop at the same rate in the permanent teeth of fluoridated and non-fluoridated children. A maximum 10-percent reduction in caries occurs in children whose teeth developed while drinking fluoridated water. While the protective effect of fluoride in caries is hotly debated, it seems to be agreed that once the permanent teeth have fully formed and emerged, high fluoride intake no longer has any effect. Adult teeth do not benefit from fluoridated water.

A comparison of cancer rates in the ten largest U.S. cities fluoridated before 1966 with rates of the ten largest cities during the prefluoride period (1944–1950), and not fluoridated as of 1969, demonstrated a significant increase in the incidence of cancer and cancer deaths in fluoridated cities. A similar study, however, detected no difference in cancer rates between fluoridated and non-fluoridated U.S. counties. The problems inherent in both studies are manifold.

Another debate centers on the possible correlation between congenital malformations and a fluoridated water supply. Schatz has reported that fluoridation of the water supply in Chilean cities increased infant mortality and congenital malformations by as much as 288 percent. On the other hand, a study in the United States of a comparison of metropolitan Atlanta to several other metropolitan areas showed no association of congenital malformations with fluoridated areas. The difference in findings may relate to the basic nutrition in each population. The Chileans of Curico are relatively malnourished, and hence would be more susceptible to the dangers of fluoride. The increased sensitivity of malnourished peoples to fluoride has resulted in an epidemic of genum valgum [knock-knees] in India.

Claims as to the role of fluoride in heart and vascular conditions have also been contradictory. Similar population studies, as above, have shown both increases and no association between water fluoridation and these conditions.

Ingesting large amounts of fluoride initially produces no observable effects. (The exact amount has not been ascertained, but the danger line is 1.5 ppm; even fluoride advocates agree that 2 ppm is toxic after twenty to fifty years.) One known effect of excessive fluoride intake in children—mottling of the tooth enamel—does not insure against dental caries, however. In both children and adults, a prompt rise in urinary fluoride excretion occurs to a maximum, and then bone deposition occurs.

Fluoride is administered in many different salt forms. In cases of bone degeneration, sodium fluoride is prescribed in doses of 1 to 50 mg a day; side effects include gastroenteritis and loss of appetite. Potassium and calcium fluoride are also sometimes prescribed. The degree of toxicity of these compounds is related to their solubility; hence, calcium is least toxic, followed by potassium and sodium compounds. In an experiment conducted by Dr. William Costain, all of his patients given 3 mg of sodium fluoride suffered ill effects. The fluoride encountered in natural drinking water is calcium fluoride; soft water contains little fluoride. U.S. water supplies are usually fluoridated by sodium fluoride, sodium silico fluoride or hydro fluorosilic acid. Large quantities of these compounds are very toxic, and silicon accumulation in brain tissue has been related to Alzheimer's disease. Thus, calcium fluoride should be the agent whenever communities decide in favor of fluoridation.

Certainly, the only reason to fluoridate a water supply is for purposes of disease prevention, and dental caries seems to represent the only near bona fide case for disease prevention. In a plot drawn between occurrence of mottling versus maximum dental caries inhibition, the two curves intersected at 1 ppm; this amount, then, is the recommended level of water fluoridation.

Community fluoridation ranges from 0.7 to 1.2 ppm. The margin for error between first signs of toxicity, 1.5 to 2 ppm, is minimal. A complicating factor in setting levels is that fluoride is cumulative at any level of intake; some fluoride poisoning has even occurred in areas where the water supply was *not* fluoridated. Moreover, individual diet and susceptibility make even 1 ppm questionable. One thing that is certain, however, is that fluoridated water makes increased mottling of teeth inevitable. It has been estimated that when a water supply is at the recommended 1 ppm level, the personal intake of fluoride increases threefold.

When food is cooked in water containing fluoride, its fluoride content increases. In Canada, ginger ale made with fluoridated water contains 0.77 ppm as compared with only 0.02 ppm for ginger ale made with non-fluoridated water. Tomato soup reconstituted with fluoridated water contains 0.38 ppm as compared to 0.4 ppm for non-fluoridated. In other words, the overall intake of fluoride does not depend solely on the concentration in the water alone but also on products made with water. Studies reveal that the water intake of individuals may vary as much as 20 to 1. When fluoride is added to water supplies, the dietary levels of fluoride become tremendously increased and varied.

Most proponents of fluoride agree that the administration of fluoride tablets to women during pregnancy and lactation, and to children is as effective as fluoridated water in decreasing dental caries. Tablet consumption achieves all the benefits claimed for fluoride, and an additional benefit is that it is four to five times less costly than fluoridating the water supply. The only problem with tablets is that it is most difficult to maintain conscientious tablet consumption on a wide scale. The topical application of fluoride is as effective as tablets—hence, the popularity of fluoridated toothpastes. (Toothpastes with calcium fluoride should be used.)

References

Bierenbaum, M. L. Effect of fluoridated water upon serum lipids, ions and cardiovascular disease, mortality rates. *J. of Med. Soc. of N.J.* 71(9):663–666, 1974.

Burgstahler, A. W., et al. Statement concerning Kansas house bill 2220. Prepared for presentation to the Committee on Public Health and Welfare, 24 February 1975.

Daniel, H. J. Fluoride and clinical otosclerosis. *Arch. Otlaryngol* 98:327–329, 1973.

Erickson, J. D. Water fluoridation and congenital malformation: no association. *JADA*, 93:981–984, 1976.

A feast of fluoride. *Emergency Medicine* 12:65, 1976.

Gotzsche, A. L. *The fluoride question: Panacea or poison?* Briarcliff Manor, N.Y., 1975, p. 176.

Griffith, H. J. The role of calcium and fluoride in osteoporosis in rhesus monkeys. *Investigative Radiology* 10(3):263–267, 1975.

Holdsworth, C. E. Comparative biochemical study of otosclerosis and ostogenesis imperfecta. *Arch. Otolaryngol* 98:335–339, 1973.

Hoover, R. N., et al. Fluoridated drinking water and the occurrence of cancer. *J. Natl. Cancer* 57(4):757–768, 1976.

House, H. P., et al. Sodium fluoride and the otosclerotic lesion. *Arch. Otolaryngol* 100:427–430, 1974.

Krishnamachari, K.A.V.R. The use of Nagarjunsager Canal water in the control of fluorosis in Andrha Pradesh—a preliminary study. *Indian J. Med. Res.* 63(3):475–479, 1975.

National Health Federation Bulletin. Delaney amendment could be death-knell to fluoridation. 19 September 1975, pp. 5–15.

Nesin, B. C. A water supply perspetive of the fluoridation discussion. Maine Water Utilities Association, 28 February 1956.

Schatz, A. The failure of fluoridation in England. *Prevention*, August 1972, pp. 64–69.

Schatz, A. Increased death rates in Chile associated with artificial fluoridation of drinking water with implications for other countries. *J. of Arts, Sciences, and Humanities* 2(1):11–16, 1976.

Schroeder, H. A. *The Trace Elements and Man.* Old Greenwich, Connecticut: Devin-Adair, 1973.

Toth, K. Optimum and tolerated intake of fluorine. *Acta Medica Academise Scientarium Hungaricae* 32(1):1–14, 1975.

Toxic effects of fluoride in enamel formation. *Nutrition Reviews* 34(10):311–313, 1976.

Underwood, E. J. *Trace elements in human and animal nutrition.* New York: Academic Press, Inc., 1977, Ch. 13, pp. 347–369.

Value of fluoride in prevention of dental caries. *JAMA* 234(3):312–313, 1975.

CHAPTER 16

Nickel:
An Essential Trace Metal
but Where?

In the 1920s the trace element nickel was discovered in animal tissues. At one time, nickel was thought to be the only element in the periodic table not essential to animals; this belief resulted from the difficulty in preparing nickel-deficient diets, since nickel is ubiquitous. (It occurs in the air, in plants and in animals, including the newborn.) Until recently, researchers were also handicapped by the lack of appropriate environments for the raising and maintaining of laboratory animals. However, nickel has been found to have a physiological role both in animal and human metabolism.

More is known about the effects of nickel in certain animals than in man. Nickel in tissues outside the intestine intensifies the hypoglycemic effect of insulin in both the rabbit and the dog. Large doses alter lipid (fatty substance) metabolism, and injection of nickel amino acid complexes into rabbits increases plasma lipids. In humans, it has an antidotal effect on the hypertensive action of adrenalin (the hormone found in the adrenal medulla area of the brain) which acts as a vasoconstrictor and cardiac stimulant. Its possible physiological function, therefore, may involve hormone, lipid and also membrane metabolism.

In human blood serum a concentration of nickel is maintained within a characteristic range. High levels may occur in patients who suffer from a blockage of blood flow to the heart (myocardial infarction), in patients with strokes and severe burns and in women with toxemia of pregnancy or uterine cancer. Low levels occur in patients with cirrhosis of the liver or chronic kidney failure. Significant concentrations of nickel are found in DNA and RNA and may contribute to the stabilization of nucleic acids.

Contradictions

Evidence concerning the potentially harmful or beneficial effects of nickel seems contradictory. Although nickel is essential in the diet of chickens, it can be toxic to humans when absorbed in large quantities. Nielsen and Sauberlich reported in 1970 that young chicks fed a regulated diet consisting of 40 ppb of nickel (high dose) developed symptoms of pigmentation changes in the shank skin, swelling in the legs, dermatitis, fat- and oxygen-depleted livers (and thus suboptimal function of that organ) and a small accumulation of nickel in the liver, bone and aorta.

The ill effects of nickel and nickel-containing compounds in humans probably range from dermatitis to lung cancer. Exposure to nickel is widespread, since it is found in such common articles as nickel coins, eyeglass frames, costume jewelry, kitchen appliances, pins, scissors and hair clips. Nickel can be most dangerous when present in combination with carbon monoxide. The resulting substance, nickel carbonyl, which is encountered in many industries, can be lethal. Recently, thirty-one men working in an oil refinery were exposed to nickel carbonyl and required hospitalization; three died as a result. Symptoms of this poisoning are frontal headache, vertigo, nausea and vomiting. Delayed reactions may also include constrictive chest pain and cough.

A final warning to cigarette smokers: nickel and its carbonyls are suspected of causing cancer, and nickel carbonyl is found in tobacco and is present in cigarette smoke. It has been shown that the amount of nickel capable of inducing lung cancer in rats is equivalent to that of fifteen cigarettes a day smoked for one year.

Nickel may be used in an organic complex, as cobalt is in vitamin B-12, or as chromium is in the glucose tolerance factor. This conjecture needs further study.

References

Nielsen, F. H. and Ollerich, D. A. Nickel: a new essential trace element. *Federation Proceedings* 33:6, June 1974.

Nielsen, F. H. and Sauberlich, H. E. Evidence of a possible requirement for nickel by the chick. *Proc. Soc. Exp. Biol. and Med.* 134:3, July 1970.

Studies show nickel could play major metabolic role. *JAMA* 214:4, 26 October 1972.

Sunderman, F. Jr.; Nomoto, S.; Pradhan, A.M.; Levine, H.; Bernstein, S. H. and Hirsch, R. Increased concentrations of serum nickel after acute myocardial infarction. *New Eng. J. of Med.* 283:896–899, 22 October 1970.

Sunderman, F. Jr.; Nomoto, S.; Morang, R.; Nechay, M. W.; Burke, C. N. and Nielsen, S. W. Nickel deprivation in chicks. *J. Nutr.* 102:259–268, February 1972.

Trace metals—medicine's newest alchemy: II, an essential role for nickel? *Medical World News*, 21 April 1972.

von Mertz, D. P., Koschnick, R. and Wilk, G. The renal excretion of nickel by humans. Studies on the metabolism of trace elements, IV. *Z. Klin. Chem. u. Klin. Biochem.* Berlin: Walter de Gruyter, 1970.

Nickel Update 1978

Biological Complexes

A nickel protein named nickeloplasmin exists in human and rabbit serum; its function in either man or animals is not as yet known.

Like zinc, nickel forms a complex with the phytate in grains which will decrease absorption. Iron forms similar structures with phytic acid with a resulting decrease in absorption.

Nickel and Disease

Rats raised on a nickel-deficient diet develop anemia, which is not corrected even by doubling the iron intake. Nickel probably assists in iron absorption in the same manner as does cobalt.

Nickel deficiency seems unlikely to arise under conditions of good nutrition.

References

Schnegg, A. and Kirchgessner, M. Zur Absorption und Verfugbarkeit von Eisen bei Nickel-Mangel. *International Journal for Vitamin and Nutrition Research* 46:96–99, 1976.

Underwood, E. J. *Trace elements in human and animal nutrition*. New York: Academic Press, 1977, Ch. 6.

CHAPTER 17

Aluminum

ALUMINUM. What is it and how is it used? If a layman were asked what aluminum is used for, he might say that it is used as foil to wrap foods and to make pots and pans. A scientist might reply that it is used in antacids, deodorants and baking powder. However, when asked what aluminum's function is in the human body, most people probably would not know. Scientists don't know either! There is still a great deal to learn about it.

Although aluminum is plentiful in the earth, relatively low concentrations are found in the tissues of plants and animals. Dr. Henry Schroeder, a foremost authority on the relationships between trace elements and man, believes that there may be more aluminum in modern man than was present in primitive man; one of the principal causes may be food additives. For example, sodium aluminum phosphate is used as an emulsifier in some processed cheeses. Table salt often contains sodium silico aluminate or aluminum calcium silicate to prevent the salt from caking. One of the bleaching agents used to whiten flour is potassium alum, an aluminum-containing compound.

The body stores its highest concentrations of aluminum in the lungs, liver, thyroid and brain. Usually, most of the aluminum taken into the body is later excreted. Although concern has been expressed about the ingestion of aluminum from cookware and aluminum-containing baking powder, some authorities such as E. J. Underwood and H. A. Schroeder contend that no harmful effects or dangers result from using these things in the preparation of food.

Dr. Schroeder discovered that mice and rats fed 10 ppm aluminum in their drinking water during their lifetime did not develop ill effects either in their growth or lifespan. Ehrismann reported in 1939 that rabbits and guinea pigs exposed to aluminum dust six hours daily for several weeks showed no abnormalities except for irritation of the lining of the nose and throat with the larger doses.

However, the stomach antacid, aluminum hydroxide gel, which has many trade names, can greatly reduce blood phosphate, according to L. R. I. Baker of London. With low serum phosphate the bones dissolve, the muscles ache and are extremely weak. In a patient on regular dialysis therapy for his poor kidney function, bone pain and the muscle weakness disappeared six weeks after the aluminum hydroxide therapy was stopped. The porosity of the bones was healed in three months, as judged by X-ray examination. Older patients, who are particularly subject to osteoporosis, should therefore limit their use of aluminum hydroxide gel.

To date, there is no conclusive evidence that aluminum is essential for the life of microorganisms, plants, animals or man. On the contrary, aluminum may be harmful.

Aluminum's Ill Effects

Many aluminum salts have antisweat effects when used with other chemicals. Because of this, many deodorants contain aluminum salts which can produce a contact dermatitis and irritation. The skin rash disappears when the deodorant is discontinued. This rash is minor compared with the possible brain damage which can result from too much inhaled or ingested aluminum.

Kopeloff et al. reported in 1942 that in animals the

application of trace amounts of aluminum to the surface of the brain will initiate the electrical activity of seizures or fits. According to Klatzo et al., the injection of aluminum salts into the fluid surrounding the brain will initiate the degeneration characteristic of some types of senile dementia. Crapper et al. at the University of Toronto have found that aluminum-injected cats are slower learners in a simple conditioned avoidance task. The level of aluminum in the cats' brains is exactly equivalent to the high level of aluminum (12 mcg per gm) found in the brains of patients suffering from Alzheimer's disease, which is one type of senile dementia. The authors point out that this comparably high level in the two instances suggests that aluminum may be a poison in human senility. Aluminum therefore may be implicated as a factor in at least one brain disease.

As investigation of the rarer trace elements opens new vistas, uncharted regions appear that need to be explored. Aluminum is a prime example. More research needs to be done on the presence of high levels of aluminum in the brains of senile individuals and epileptics. In the meantime, aluminum pans should not be cleaned by cooking acid fruits, such as rhubarb, in them. The cleaning water goes into the rhubarb and hence into the unsuspecting consumer.

References

Adams, R. and Murray, F. *Minerals: Kill or cure?* New York: Larchmont Books, 1974.

Baker, L. R. I. et al. *Br. Med. J.* 3:150–151, 20 July 1974.

Crapper, D. R., Krishman, S. S. and Dalton, A. J. Brain aluminum distribution and experimental neuro-fibrillary degeneration. *Science* 180, May 1973.

Furia, T. E. *Handbook of food additives.* Cleveland; The Chemical Rubber Co., 1968.

Klatzo, I., Wisniewski, E. and Streicher, J. *J. Neuropathol. Exp. Neurol.* 23:187, 1965.

Kopeloff, L., Barrera, S. and Kopeloff, N. *Amer. J. Psychiat.* 98:881, 1942.

McLaughlin, A. I. G.; Kazantzis, G.; King, E.; Teare, D.; Porter, R. J. and Owen, R. *Brit. J. Ind. Med.* 19:253, 1962.

Schroeder, H. A. *The trace elements and man.* Old Greenwich, Connecticut: Devin-Adair, 1973.

Sollman, T., *A manual of pharmacology.* 8th ed. Philadelphia: W. B. Saunders, 1957.

Underwood, E. J., *Trace elements in human and animal nutrition.* London: Academic Press, 1971.

Aluminum Update 1978

Aluminum is present in all human tissues. In small amounts it can enhance and inhibit specific enzymes, but in larger quantities it can be toxic. Aluminum is a component of buffered aspirin, antacids, toothpastes, baking powders, cooking utensils, dental amalgams, prostheses (artificial parts), cigarette filters, food additives, food wrappers and cosmetics. As a flocculent it is added to our drinking water in the form of sulfate. It is most extensively used as an ingredient in phosphate binding gels.

Aluminum Encephalopathy

Aluminum binding products (Amphojel, Gelusel, and the like) are widely used to control serum phosphate levels in kidney patients on dialysis. There have been thirty-one cases recognized of total loss of brain function linked to aluminum intoxication in patients ingesting aluminum gels, 4 grams a day (1 gram of aluminum per day). Patients first suffer progressive speech difficulties, then memory loss and finally total mental lethargy, becoming human vegetables. These symptoms are not always constant, but at least a seven-month deterioration period occurs before death. Attempts to reverse the syndrome can be initiated by stopping aluminum hydroxide (the major ingredient of gels), but in spite of all such therapy death occurs in about one year. Possibly some reversal can be achieved by withdrawing the aluminum hydroxide and adding phosphate. Apparently, the encephalopathy is partly a result of phosphate depletion caused by excess aluminum. The use of a chelator EDTR has been successful in reversing the encephalopathy. Autopsies on victims confirm that muscle, bone and the grey matter of the brain have high aluminum content (Table 17.1). To prevent aluminum poisoning, it has been suggested that magnesium hydroxide be used as a replacement for aluminum to remove excess phosphate in kidney patients.

TABLE 17.1

Aluminum levels at autopsy

Aluminum in controls (13) mg/kg dry wt.	Dialysis encephalopathy (10)
Muscle	1.22 ± 0.02	23.6 ± 18.6
Cortical bone	3.9 ± 1.7	46.8 ± 41.2
Trabecular bone	2.4 ± 1.2	98.5 ± 60.0
Brain grey	$2.2 \pm .69$	25.0 ± 9.8
Brain white	$2.0 \pm .63$	5.6 ± 1.9

Aluminum gels are not the only examples of toxicity caused by aluminum. A machine operator who worked in an aluminum flake powder factory for seventeen years developed a similar encephalopathy. In England, two deaths have been linked to aluminum-contaminated water from a hot water heater. (Such cases are not known in the United States inasmuch as in England an aluminum metal cathode is used in hot water heaters to prevent corrosion, whereas magnesium is used in the United States.) Another form of aluminum toxicity is permanent skin discoloring resulting from close contact with rubbing compounds used to polish aluminum cookware. Aluminum products also slow down the rate and extent of absorption of tetracycline

TABLE 17.2
Aluminum blood levels in patients with pre-senile dementia

	Control Group	Pre-senile* Dementia	
n = Number of patients	n = 20	n = 16	
Age	59.0 ± 10.9 yrs.**	59.3 ± 9.8 yrs.	t = 0.088 N.S.
Aluminum (Whole blood)	2.6 ± 1.4 mcg/%	6.6 ± 6.8 mcg/%	t = 2.6 p <0.05
Manganese (Whole blood)	1.5 ± 0.5 mcg/%	1.3 ± 0.4 mcg/%	t = 1.9 N.S.
Copper (Serum)	118.3 ± 13.8 mcg/%	128.6 ± 17.8 mcg/%	t = 1.2 N.S.
Lead (Whole blood)	14.3 ± 3.9 mcg/% (n = 17)	14.2 ± 3.0 mcg/% (n = 10)	t = 0.05 N.S.

* Patients exhibiting loss of memory, loss of concentration and confusion.
** Mean ± S.D.
N.S. = Not significant
SOURCE: Data of Dr. Arthur Sohler, Ph.D.

antibiotics. Aluminum absorption occurs in all human beings exposed to a source of aluminum. In normal human beings, excess aluminum actually results in elevated serum phosphorus due to an interaction that is not present in dialysis patients.

Senile Dementia

Alzheimer's disease or pre-senile dementia causes more deaths annually than cancer. Starting in mid-adult life the victim exhibits loss of memory for recent events (Table 17.2—BBC data). Patients who die as a result of this disease have always had brain neurofibrillary tangles, cell degeneration and too much aluminum and silicon in the brain and cerebrospinal fluid. The neurofibrillary tangles have been associated with aluminum poisoning in many common laboratory animals. The same changes occur locally if aluminum is applied to the exposed surface of the brain. Despite minor discrepancies in reports as to the location of the excess aluminum in the brain, aluminum seems to be a major factor in Alzheimer's disease. Intoxication by lead and other metals or zinc deficiency may be other causes of pre-senile dementia.

What Level in Drinking Water?

Millions of pounds of aluminum sulfate are used to purify drinking water systems every year. The substance, an efficient precipitant that forms filterable clumps with impurities, is highly soluble in water, and we know that all the aluminum is not filtered out. High aluminum content in the water of South Wales in Australia has been linked positively to congenital malformations of the central nervous system (Table 17.3). Unfortunately, public health or Environmental Protection Agency water standards for aluminum do not exist; therefore, aluminum content in tap water can vary considerably in all areas of the country.

TABLE 17.3

Aluminum and other metals in water supply of South Wales, Australia, correlated with birth defects

Metal	No. of Samples	AM	Correl Coef.	PM	Correl Coef.
Calcium	48	25.6	−0.30	25.2	−0.31
Magnesium	48	5.2	−0.15	5.1	−0.13
Manganese	48	0.023	+0.21	0.014	−0.04
Copper	48	0.26	−0.42	0.11	−0.38
Zinc	48	0.203	−0.14	0.086	−0.09
Aluminum	48	0.061	+0.30	0.49	+0.31

Samples are from forty-eight different communities in South Wales. Only aluminum has a positive correlation with birth defects for all samples. Copper and calcium may help prevent birth defects.

The toxic effect of aluminum has not been studied carefully since the introduction of aluminum baking powders in the 1920s. Since 1920, the use of aluminum and its salts in the water, food, drug and cookware industries has increased to the point where we may lose our minds prematurely. The time has come for all consumers to read labels and to avoid city water, free flowing salt, buffered aspirin, antacids, toothpastes, baking powders and cooking utensils that contain aluminum.

References

Alfrey, A. L., et al. The dialysis encephalopathy syndrome. *New England Journal of Medicine* 294:184–188, 1976.

Burks, J. S., et al. A fatal encephalopathy in chronic hemodialysis patients. *The Lancet* 4/10:764–768, 1976.

Cam, J. M., et al. The effect of aluminum hydroxide orally on calcium, phosphorus, and aluminum metabolism in normal subjects. *Clinical Science and Molecular Medicine* 51:407–414, 1976.

De Boni, V., et al. Neurofibrillary degeneration induced by systemic aluminum. *Acta Neuropath* 35:285–294, 1976.

Duckett, S., et al. Mise en evidence de l'aluminum dans les plaques saniles de la maladie d'Alzheimer. *C. R. Acad. Sci.* 282:393, 1976.

Flendrig, J. A., et al. Aluminum and dialysis dementia. *The Lancet* 6/5:1235, 1976.

Guirard, B. M., et al. Vitamin B–6 function in transamination and decarboxylation. *Comprehensive biochemistry*, edited by M. F. Lorkin, et al. New York, 1964, p. 15.

Harrison, W. H., et al. Aluminum inhibition of hexokinase. *The Lancet* 2:277, 1972.

Lynch, J. D. Skin discoloration from buffing compounds on aluminum cookware. *JAMA* 235(26):2875, 1976.

Morton, M. S., et al. Trace elements in water and congenital malformations of the central nervous system in South Wales. *Br. J. of Preventive and Social Med.* 30(1): 36–39, 1976.

Pieridedes, A. M., et al. Hemodialysis encephalopathy: possible role of phosphate depletion. *The Lancet* 6/5:1234–1235, 1976.

Possible aluminum intoxication. *Nutrition Reviews* 34(6):166–167, 1976.

Sorenson, J. R. J., et al. Aluminum in the environment and human health. *Environmental Health Perspectives* 8:3–95, 1974.

CHAPTER 18

Lead, Mercury and Cadmium

Lead Poisoning

INVESTIGATORS are now busy assessing the role of lead and methyl mercury in hyperactivity and mental retardation in children and poisoned animals. To date, most of the available data are on lead poisoning. The pioneer article appeared in *Lancet* in 1972. Dr. Oliver David and his colleagues at the Downstate Medical Center in Brooklyn set up a study which employed a challenging dose of penicillamine in three groups of children. Penicillamine, a chelating agent, promotes the excretion of lead via the urinary pathway. The first group of children in the study were known to have been lead poisoned, the second were hyperactive children and the third were "normal" children. The individuals of each group were challenged with a 500 mg. dose of penicillamine at bedtime and the morning urine was collected from each child. The lead level in the urine was determined under blind test conditions. The excretion of lead was highest (325 micrograms per liter—mcg/1) in those children diagnosed as lead poisoned but in remission. The next highest urinary lead excretion was in the hyperactive children (146 mcg/1) and their lead excretion was significantly different from that of the "normal" children (77 mcg/1). All children were from poorer sections of Brooklyn and had been exposed daily to the usual hazards of lead intoxication from auto exhaust and old paint dust.

Drs. Michaelson and Sauerhoff of Cincinnati fed 4 percent lead carbonate to rats and found that the animals became hyperactive. Drs. Silbergelb and Goldberg of Johns Hopkins in Baltimore fed mice lead and again found hyperactivity. This abnormal activity was reduced by deanol or amphetamine therapy and made worse by phenobarbitol, a correlation with the known drug response in hyperactive children. Others have studied the effect of lead in rhesus monkeys and very young baboons. However, the degree of hyperactivity in these larger species was not measured.

Finally, Drs. Niklowitz and Yeager of Cincinnati have exposed rats to tetraethyl lead and analyzed the brains for levels of the more common trace elements zinc, copper and iron. All three of these essential trace elements were significantly decreased by lead exposure. Results of the study strongly indicate that the specific toxic property of lead which causes abnormal brain function is its ability to interfere competitively with the trace metal components of zinc, copper and iron dependent enzymes which regulate mental processes.

Auto Exhaust Lead

Many sources of lead in the environment are potentially hazardous. A major source of environmental lead is pollution from auto exhaust. Tetraethyl lead is added to most high-test gasolines to improve acceleration and as an antiknock. The concentration of lead in the atmosphere of large cities and in the air near interstate highways is so high as to cause toxic reactions in some particularly toxicity-prone individuals. Toll booth collectors have been known to exhibit toxic blood levels of lead. Caprio and his colleagues at the New Jersey College of Medicine in Newark studied inner-city children who lived near arterial highways. They found blood lead levels to be higher in children who lived closest to these roads. Many of the children had lead levels above 60 mcg percent—a level which indicates lead poisoning.

Darrow and his colleagues at Brattleboro, Vermont have found that sweepings from parking lots are sufficiently high in heavy metals as to retard the growth of young animals when these sweepings are added to the diet. The most likely poison from parking lots is lead from auto exhaust. Lead also often appears in the vegetation beside well-travelled highways. Cows who subsist on this vegetation alone can have lead-induced abortions. Vegetables grown beside busy highways should not be eaten unless their lead content can be proven safe for consumption.

The latest in a long series of smelter pollutions has occurred in Kellogg, Idaho where the Bunker Hill zinc smelter may have polluted the downwind environment with lead dust. Some of the children of Kellogg have developed lead poisoning for no apparent cause. Houses closest to the smelter had more children with lead poisoning. While the smelter may not be entirely to blame, the cumulative effect of smelter lead and auto exhaust lead can add up to clinical lead poisoning. When discovered, such communities should be labeled disaster areas with funds available for cleaning or relocation of homes and other buildings.

Lead may also enter our ambient air through cigarettes, due to the lead arsenate applied to the tobacco as an insecticide, through the burning of coal, and through the fumes and ash produced by the burning of lead battery casings. The decay products of gaseous radon, which enter the atmosphere through natural volcanic activity, contribute to the lead content of ambient air. At present, however, the chief source is exhaust from autos burning leaded gasoline.

In urban areas, the concentration of lead in polluted air varies inversely with altitude. This is only logical since lead is such a heavy element. Consequently, we find that lead poisoning occurs frequently in small urban dogs. Epilepsy is usually the first symptom. Unfortunately, it is also frequent among young urban people who toddle about close to the ground. In these, hyperactivity may be the first presenting symptom.

Lead in Water: Mental Retardation

Another dangerous environmental source of lead is from the drinking water in soft water regions which courses through lead plumbing systems. Soft water is more acidic than hard water. Because of its acidity, soft water will erode lead from lead piping and become contaminated with this heavy metal.

A group of investigators in Glasgow, Scotland, directed by Dr. A. D. Beattie of Stobhill Hospital, have established a significant correlation between lead ingested from contaminated soft drinking water and mental retardation in children. Dr. Beattie and his team studied 154 Glasgow children. Seventy-seven of the children were attending clinics in Glasgow because of retardation in mental development while the remaining seventy-seven were nonretarded healthy youngsters forming a control group matched for age, sex and geographic location in the city.

The investigators collected water samples from the taps of the homes where the children lived and also collected blood samples from their subjects. Analysis of the samples revealed significantly greater amounts of lead in water from the homes of the retarded children as compared with that from the homes of the normal children. Blood levels of lead were also higher in the retarded group than in the control group, strongly implicating tap water lead as the cause of brain damage.

Dr. Beattie and his colleagues further postulate that tap water lead poses a serious threat to children even before birth. Lead ingested by mothers drinking contaminated tap water is capable of crossing the placenta to the fetus. Since the blood-brain barrier in the fetus is less developed and therefore more permeable to toxic substances than it is in the full-term infant, the prenatal hazards of lead poisoning would indeed be probable.

On the basis of their findings, Dr. Beattie and his

team emphasize the need to remove lead from plumbing systems (e.g. water tanks and pipes). Although this would be the most satisfactory solution, several years will be required to accomplish this goal. In the meantime, water reservoirs supplying Glasgow will be treated with calcium salts. By decreasing the acidity of the soft water, calcium salts will protect the water supplies from lead contamination.

Calcium versus Lead

Furthermore, sufficient dietary calcium has been found effective in preventing the accumulation of lead in body tissues. Two researchers, K. M. Six and R. A. Goyer, discovered that reducing dietary calcium in rats greatly enhanced the body burden of lead as evidenced by increased levels of lead in blood, bone and soft tissues. Professor C. Snowden of the University of Wisconsin also found that in calcium-deficient rats given water containing lead, lead replaced the lacking calcium in bones and teeth. Experimental studies conducted by L. G. Lederer and F. C. Bing, again using rats, indicated that adequate dietary calcium prevents accumulation of lead in body tissues by reducing absorption of ingested lead from the intestinal tract, a finding supported by the research of Professor F. Hsu and his colleagues at Cornell University using weanling pigs. Since calcium protects both water and body tissues from lead contamination, the addition of this trace element to drinking water supplies in high risk areas such as Glasgow will be highly beneficial.

Lead in Paint

Lead-based paints are another source of lead poisoning. A New York psychiatrist, Dr. William Niederland, speculates that a mysterious mental illness which struck the Spanish painter Goya at the age of 46, was lead poisoning caused by the artist's use of lead-based paints. For years, art historians have considered this illness to be the cause of an abrupt change in the subject matter of Goya's work—from pleasant court portraiture to grotesque social commentary. Dr. Niederland points out that Goya used large quantities of white paint made from lead carbonate in his work and, unlike other painters, often completed an entire painting in a single afternoon. Lead carbonate will seep through the intact skin and also give off noxious vapors. As a result of consistent and prolonged periods of exposure to a toxic lead compound, Goya would have absorbed into his bloodstream amounts of lead sufficient to produce brain damage. According to Dr. Niederland, the symptoms of Goya's illness—vertigo, mental confusion, hallucinations and impaired balance, hearing and speech—are characteristic of fulminating lead encephalopathy.

Three- or four-year-olds who cut their milk teeth on peeling lead-based paint or plaster in old dilapidated housing frequently develop lead poisoning. School children who chew on the lead-containing paint coatings of pencils can develop lead poisoning. Adults who attempt to remove old lead-based paint by the usual dusty mechanical methods can also get lead poisoning—only wet methods should be used.

Lead: Pottery

The home craftsman (or woman) should be especially careful of certain lead-containing pottery glazes. If fired at too low a temperature, the lead in the glaze is not fixed and can leach out into foods.

Your children are highly susceptible to lead poisoning from a wide variety of sources. Pica—the consumption of such items as dirt, paper and paint, all of which contain lead—is often the cause of lead intoxication in youngsters. Even babies, who are not yet subject to the range of exposure possible with mobility, are not safe. The lead plugs used to seal evaporated milk cans are an occasional source of lead for infant formulas. Lead seams of fruit juice cans are a more frequent source.

Lead: Pet Food

Pet owners who dote on their precious furry friends
might well become enraged at the news that poor Fido
may be consuming toxic amounts of lead in his canned
dog food. Others, less concerned with the welfare of
the animal population, might simply shrug and say,
"Well, I'm glad I don't eat dog food!" until acquainted
with the full implications of this recent discovery. Researchers Hankin and Heichel of the Connecticut Agricultural Experiment Station, who determined that
canned pet foods contain as much as 5.6 ppm lead,
traced the lead contamination of such products to the
processed organ meats which constitute the main ingredient of Fido's feed. With a daily ingestion of 170 gm
(6 oz.) pet foods could contribute up to 1.19 mg of
lead to the animal or human diet—about four times the
dose of lead (0.3 mg per day) potentially toxic for
children. Still convinced that only Fido faces the danger of lead poisoning, one must recall that humans,
too, consume processed and fresh organ meats, Liver,
for example, is a principal constituent of liverwurst,
sausage and popular sandwich spreads. Upon examining seven samples of commercial liverwurst, Hankin
and Heichel found lead levels ranging between 1.8 and
7.6 ppm. On the basis of a daily consumption of 113
gm (4 oz.) these products could contribute 0.20 to
0.86 mg lead to the human diet—about 0.6 to 2.9
times the dose of lead potentially toxic for children.
Market samples of fresh beef and pork liver examined
by the two researchers showed lead levels ranging between 1.4 and 1.6 ppm and levels as high as 5.6 ppm
in pork, 7.6 ppm in beef and 10.9 ppm in turkey have
been reported. Such meats, then, would contribute even
greater quantities of lead to the human diet. On the
basis of these findings, fresh liver sausage would be a
doubly hazardous food. Farmers may supplement their
hogs' feed with copper sulfate in order to accelerate the
animals' weight gain. Copper, like lead, is a toxic

heavy metal and liver already contains lead, so the poor sausage-lover is threatened on two counts!

Thus, even though most people do not consume pet food, liver and other organ meats are normal components of the human diet and the inadvertent ingestion of lead (and copper) by humans eating liver products is yet another insidious environmental source of heavy metal poisoning.

Because of increasing evidence linking excess blood and tissue lead with hyperactivity and mental retardation, researchers have sought simple, valid methods for determining the presence of toxic amounts of lead in the body. Although it is possible, direct analysis of blood for lead, which demands expensive equipment, skill in analytical technique and great care to avoid the risk of sample contamination from environmental lead, is unsuitable as a general diagnostic procedure.

Simple Test

Recently, Dr. A. A. Lamola and his colleagues at the Bell Laboratories in New Jersey successfully devised a simple, inexpensive diagnostic screening test for lead poisoning. Together with his coworkers, Dr. Lamola found that the metabolite zinc protoporphyrin (ZPP) accumulates in erythrocytes (red blood cells) as a result of lead interference with heme synthesis. ZPP is a fluorescent compound which can be measured directly and accurately by means of a spectrofluorometer, thereby offering a valid indirect means of monitoring blood lead concentration. Bell Laboratories has designed a small inexpensive fluorometer which is currently undergoing field testing. If approved for use, this instrument will allow frequent examination of children in high risk populations, thus increasing the public health benefits of this new test.

The Mercury Threat

Pesticides and some large fish are the most notorious sources of mercury. If fish are poisoned by mercury, the extent of poisoning is directly proportional to the size of the fish, and therefore the large tuna such as yellow fin and big eye will then be much more likely to poison people who eat them daily than albacore or skipjack. The mercury menace in swordfish is enough to keep this large fish off the market. Swordfish used for commercial meat weigh as much as one hundred pounds.

The process known as organic complexing is responsible for the spread of the culprit compound, methyl mercury, throughout the aquatic world. Mercury-containing bacteria are first consumed by algae, and eventually the fish eat the algae and men eat the fish. At each step upward on the food chain, the concentration of methyl mercury increases. The amount of poison concentrated in the fish is thousands of times the amount concentrated in the algae. This is due to a half-life retention of mercury in fish of 200 days (i.e, every 200 days, a total of one-half the previous amount of mercury is dissipated). Fish balance their mercury with a higher level of selenium than man. Mercury selenide is not toxic because it is excreted.

Mercury enters rivers and lakes in a number of ways. Chemical companies use it as an electrode in the production of chlorine and it ends up in places like Lake St. Clair (which is closed to commercial fishing) where a large company has a chloralkali factory at Sarnia, Ontario. Paper pulp mills use mercury compounds as slimicides in their paper-making process. (Slimicides inhibit the growth of slime molds.) In 1970, the U.S. government urged fishermen not to eat or sell fish caught in Lakes Erie, Ontario, and Champlain and the Oswego and Niagara Rivers, because of the mercury threat.

Methyl Mercury and Fungicides

Accounts of mercury poisoning have appeared throughout history, dating back to the time of Hippocrates. In 1700, Ramazzini recorded mercury poisoning in surgeons using mercurial ointment. But it was not until the Minimata Bay disaster in Japan (1953–60) that the mercury content of foods was considered a serious problem. In that disaster, 111 persons died or were severely disabled after eating fish which had been contaminated with a methyl mercury-containing effluent from a local plastics factory.

Among the most striking case histories in recent times is that of the New Mexican laborer who fed seed grain sweepings to his hogs. The grain had been treated with Panogen, an organic mercury-containing antifungal agent; the hogs were eventually butchered and fed to the laborer's family. Within two weeks three out of the family of ten were stricken with a derangement of the brain and spinal cord. One girl lay unconscious for eight months in the hospital before waking totally blind and unable to speak. Her sister could walk and talk with effort, but the younger brother tumbled into a four month coma. The problem was eventually traced back to the organic mercury compound used as a fungicide. This mercury compound had passed into the hogs and the pork poisoned the family!

The use of mercurial fungicides on seed grains has caused numerous poisonings around the world. Frequently the poison warning on the side of the sack is only in English. A hungry Asiatic is not apt to take lessons in English in order to learn the meaning of words on a sack of potential food.

Ubiquitous Mercury

Mercury can accidentally originate from a variety of sources such as electric batteries, mercury vapor lamps, mercury switches and coal burning. Mercury from all coal-burning sources amounts to 3,000 metric tons per year, whereas natural sources of weathering rock and soil contribute 230 metric tons per year. Other sources include accidental breaking of thermometer and barometer bulbs and silvering pennies.

Calomel as Medicine

Calomel (mercurous chloride), widely acclaimed during the nineteenth century as the "Samson of the *Materia Medica*" due to its alleged effectiveness in the treatment of every infectious disease from smallpox to malaria, typhoid fever and even rheumatism, acts as a most insidious cause of mercury poisoning. As early as 1825, a poem appeared in a Virginia publication depicting the dire consequences of mercury poisoning which resulted from the use of this chemical and urging physicians to stop using calomel:

> How'er their patients do complain
> Of head, or heart, or nerve or vein,
> Of fever, thirst, or temper fell,
> The Medicine still is Calomel.
> Since Calomel's become their boast,
> How many patients have they lost,
> How many thousands they make ill,
> Of poison with their Calomel.

Since in recent times, calomel's laxative properties have rendered it an active ingredient in several commercial remedies, the threat of mercury poisoning remains. Dr. J. R. Wands and his colleagues have found that continued use of "insoluble" mercurous chloride as a laxative will result in severe poisoning. In two patients with chronic kidney failure, tremor, watery diarrhea and dementia who finally died, autopsy revealed exceedingly high levels of mercury in both the colon and kidney. Mercury levels above normal were found in all organs tested including the brain.

Damage due to orally administered mercurous compounds became apparent when it was discovered that acrodynia (pink disease), a once-common disease of young children, was due to the use of teething powders containing calomel. In spite of the recognition of these hazards, mercurous chloride can still be purchased over the counter.

It is clear that man, like experimental animals, can absorb mercury from the intestine when it is ingested as mercurous chloride. Mercury accumulates within the brain, preferentially located in certain neuronal populations. Eventually, it reaches concentrations that damage neural elements, resulting in a variety of clinical manifestations. Mercurous compounds taken by mouth must therefore be considered potentially toxic.

Mercury in Industry

Industrial workers are exposed to mercury in the manufacture of thermometers, mercury-arc rectifiers and other scientific equipment, the manufacture of dry cells, and the cleaning and packing of mercury compounds. Dental workers are exposed to the dangers of mercury in mercury-amalgam fillings, which contaminate the hands and atmosphere. Finally, travellers on their way to the Aland Islands might make a travel note to beware of the mercury-containing goosander eggs.

Early Diagnosis and Treatment Needed

Mercury poisoning can be helped if treated quickly with a chelating agent such as penicillamine. Approximately 10 percent of ingested mercury goes to the brain. In the cases of methyl and phenyl mercury, the brain may be quickly depleted of its zinc. Methyl mercury can cause neurotoxic effects and produce birth and genetic defects; it can produce excessive salivation, loss of teeth, gross tremor, and serious mental disturbance (e.g. "the mad hatters"). As the endpoint of its deleterious effects, overt neurological impairment or death may occur. Organic mercury compounds may irritate the skin, cause redness, irritation and blistering. Skerfring, Hanson and Lindsten (in 1970) found chromosome damage in humans exposed to mercury through consumption of mercury-poisoned fish.

The Cadmium Hazard

A third heavy metal scourge is cadmium. Sources of cadmium include refined foods which may have low zinc-to-cadmium ratios, water and mains and pipes (which may have cadmium content due to the impurities in zinc used many years ago for the galvanizing process, and through which soft water flows), coal burning and tobacco smoke. As we have seen, the outbreak of "Ouch Ouch disease" in Japan was due to cadmium, which appeared as a byproduct in the zinc-refining process.

While an excess of zinc in the body might prevent the accumulation of cadmium, a slight zinc deficiency would enhance cadmium poisoning. Cadmium can replace zinc in the body and cause high blood pressure and cardiovascular disease. Cadmium can interfere with copper metabolism as well.

Cadmium poisoning is a most subtle metal poisoning—probably only exceeded in subtlety by poisoning caused by the trace metals copper and iron. Cadmium deposits in the kidney and arteries raise blood pressure and cause early atherosclerosis. The early zinc used for galvanizing contained cadmium as an impurity. In many old buildings the big galvanized cold water tank was placed in the basement as the building was under construction. After thirty years the tanks start to leak and must be removed. The only possible method of removal is to cut the tank into smaller sections with an oxyacetylene burning torch. Basements are not noted for ventilation, and fresh air masks are seldom available. The tank cutter gets fume fever because of the zinc and cadmium. Since workers know of the discomfort, it usually falls to the lot of the biggest and bravest man to face the danger. In a state hospital system the chief engineer was the one who cut up the tanks in the old buildings and he, in due course, died of hypertension and atherosclerosis of the spinal artery. In cutting down the abandoned elevated line in New York, workers who did not wear their fresh air masks got lead poisoning from old paint.

Those who live downwind from ˘zinc smelters may be exposed to great excesses of cadmium both from air and contaminated soil. Measures are now being taken to prevent atmospheric pollution in the smelting of zinc ore.

The cigarette smoker gets cadmium from each cigarette often in sufficient quantity to produce emphysema—a disease in which the lungs have lost their natural elasticity. Patients with emphysema should stop smoking and take dietary supplements of zinc and vitamin B-6.

Trace metals have always occurred in man's natural environment. Consequently, they have played a role in our evolution and many of them are essential in our diet. However, when man began to use metals in manufacturing, the exposure to heavy metals greatly increased. In the four thousand, five hundred years since the introduction of metals in industry, there has not been time for our biological systems to adjust to more than the trace amounts formerly found.

The elements which are toxic are those which accumulate in mammalian tissue as a body burden with age. Other industrially used metal contaminants we have not discussed are: beryllium, silver, antimony, tellurium, barium and gold.

To summarize, heavy metal intoxication of the brain can cause hyperactivity in animals and presumably in some children. This hyperactivity in rats may be accompanied by a displacement of a sedative metal such as zinc from the brain. We know that zinc will antagonize mercury toxicity. Perhaps adequate zinc therapy along with chelators for lead will decrease the behavioral hyperactivity in children caused by lead toxicity. Since of hyperactivity in children, each with its own logical we will probably find in the future many other causes of hyperactivity in children, each with its own logical treatment. In the meantime, analysis for suspected lead poisoning is indicated in the hyperactive child.

TABLE 18.1

Hazardous environmental heavy metals

Metal	Sources	Illness
Lead	Auto exhaust Lead-based paints Smelter pollution Lead water pipes Lead batteries	Anemia Colic Fatigue Convulsions Hyperactivity Psychosis
Mercury	Coal burning Batteries Some fungicides Fish	Psychosis Blindness Paralysis Convulsions Kidney damage
Cadmium	Zinc smelters Cadmium plating Cigarette smoking	Hypertension Kidney damage Atherosclerosis
Copper	Acid well water Soft drink dispensers Algicide use in reservoirs Hemodialysis	Hyperactivity Psychosis Depression Disperceptions Atherosclerosis Hypertension

References

Beattie, A. D. et al. Role of chronic low-level lead exposure in the etiology of mental retardation. *Lancet* p. 589, 15 March 1975.

Caprio, R. J., Margulis, H. L. and Joselow, M. M. Lead absorption in children in relationship to urban traffic densities. *Arch. Environ. Health* 28:195, 1974.

David, L. E. et al. *Arch. Neurol.* 30:428, 1974.

David, O. et al. *Lancet* 2:900, 1972.

Environmental health perspectives. *Experimental Issue 7*, May 1974.

Fellows, L. Color pages in magazines cited as a source of lead poisoning. *The New York Times,* 25 November 1973.

Goldwater, L. J. Mercury in the environment. *Scientific American*, May 1971.

Hankin, L., Heichel, G. H. and Botsford, R. A. Lead in pet food and processed organ meats: a human problem? *JAMA* 231:484–485, 1975.

Hsu, F. et al. Interaction of dietary calcium with toxic levels of lead and zinc in pigs. *J. Nutr.* 105:112–118, 1975.

Lamola, A. A. et al. Zinc protoporphyrin (ZPP): a simple, sensitive fluorometric screening test for lead poisoning. *Clin. Chem.* 21:93–97, 1975.

Lederer, L. G. and Bing, F. C. Effect of calcium and phosphorous on retention of lead by growing organs. *JAMA* 114:1 457–2461, 1940.

Michaelson, A. and Sauerhoff, M. Hyperactivity and brain catecholamines in lead-exposed developing rats. *Science* 182:725–727, 1973.

Newman, B. Handicraft hazards: pottery made at home can be very harmful. *Wall Street Journal*, 11 November 1971.

Niklowitz, W. J. and Yeager, D. W. Interference of Pb with essential brain tissue Cu, Fe and Zn as main determinant in experimental tetraethyllead encephalopathy. *Life Sciences* 13:897–905, 1973.

Rensberger, B. Goya grotesquery laid to lead's use. *The New York Times*, 28 February 1974.

Risse, G. B. Calomel and the American medical sects during the 19th century. *Mayo Con. Proc.* 48:59, 1973.

Schroeder, H. A. Trace elements in the human environment. *The Ecologist*, May 1971.

Silbergelb, E. K. and Goldberg, A. M. A lead-induced behavioral disorder. *Life Sciences* 13:1275, 1973.

Six, K. M. and Goyer, R. A. Experimental enchancement of lead toxicity by low dietary calcium. *J. Lab Clin. Med.* 76:933–942, 1970.

Skerfring, S., Hanson, K. and Lindsten, J. *Arch. Environ. Health* 21:133, 1970.

Trace metals: unknown, unseen pollution threat. *Chemical and Engineering News,* 19 July 1971.

Wands, J. R. et al. Massachusetts General Hospital, Boston, 57:92–101, 1974.

Lead Update 1978

This update on lead is authoritative and timely since the Brain Bio Center has been actively engaged in lead research in man for the past five years. Every new patient at the Center gets a blood lead determination to ascertain whether a serious intoxication exists. We believe firmly that an abnormal metal burden, whether it be copper, lead, cadmium, mercury, silver, bismuth or aluminum, will produce aging and will shorten human life. If possible, the abnormal burden should be recognized and reduced. We consider any blood lead level above 25 mcg percent in the adult and any lead level higher than the age of the child to be an abnormal burden. Six percent of psychiatric adult patients have a blood lead level above 25 mcg percent and one-half of hyperactive children have a lead level above their age. If the serum uric acid level of children is high, this confirms that lead is high enough to affect the kidneys and to decrease the excretion of uric acid. Both excess copper and abnormal lead burdens can be reduced by a dietary supplement of zinc and 2 grams of vitamin C a day.

Lead can make the shortened life span of the poisoned adult a torment since the patient may have any combination of rheumatoid arthritis, depression, anemia, colic and continuous malaise as a result of the abnormal lead burden. The poisoned child will be mentally retarded, hyperactive and autistic, and even have convulsions. A child is more susceptible to lead poisoning than an adult simply because a child's blood brain barrier has not had time to mature and thus more of the poisonous lead goes to the brain. Since lead is synergistic with copper, this combination is more apt to be the general cause of most hyperactivity or autism in children.

Lead and Hyperactivity

The sensitivity of the central nervous system to abnormal metal intoxication is well established for lead. Several studies have suggested a relationship between asymptomatic lead exposure and deficits in perceptual and behavioral function. Lead has recently been implicated in cases of hyperactivity among children in Brooklyn, New York, and mental retardation among children in Scotland. Dr. Oliver David of Brooklyn has reported a study in which urinary lead excretion after the administration of penicillamine was measured in three groups of children from a center city environment. Lead excretion was highest in the group diagnosed as lead poisoned, but a group of hyperactive children also excreted significantly higher amounts of lead compared to that excreted by the third group, the normal controls.

Hyperactivity has been induced in rats by feeding them lead salts. This hyperactivity responds to amphetamines and deanol but is worsened by phenobarbital—exactly as happens in children.

Lead and Mental Retardation

In a study by Beattie, et al., in Glasgow, Scotland, a relationship was found between lead levels in the water supply and mental retardation. The houses of the affected subjects in Beattie's study were found to have lead piping from the water main to the house; another precipitating factor was that Glasgow has soft water from reservoirs (the softer the water, the greater degree of erosion of the lead plumbing). The retarded children also had higher blood lead levels than non-related matched controls. Large U.S. cities that may also have lead piping from the water mains to homes are Boston, Providence, Philadelphia, New York and Baltimore. Even small towns such as Bennington, Vermont, have occasional cases of lead poisoning in both dogs and man because of lead piping, leaded gasoline and leaded newsprint. Dr. Oliver David has found that children classified as mental retardates also have appreciable levels of lead, thus confirming Beattie's findings in Scotland.

Psychiatric Symptoms from Lead

Lead intoxication can produce many psychiatric symptoms. In cases of poisoning by tetraethyl lead, excitement, restlessness, insomnia, nightmares, hallucinations, impairment of memory and loss of mental concentration are reported. In inorganic lead poisoning, severe mental depression is often the most important symptom. Drs. Harriman and Parland have reported that industrial workers exposed to lead, while showing no obvious signs of lead poisoning, exhibit intellectual disturbances, personality changes and impaired performance in psychometric tests. While all such information is in the literature and free for the reading, doctors who see mental patients seldom suspect lead and usually do not know how or when to diagnose lead poisoning.

Vitamin C Antidotes for Heavy Metals

Vitamin C or ascorbic acid is known to have a measurable effect on both the essential trace metals and the toxic heavy metals. Under physiological conditions, vitamin C acts as a strong reducing agent to bind metal ions and affect their movement across biological membranes. Dr. Spivey Fox has shown that the addition of vitamin C to the diet of the Japanese quail reduces the toxicity of a diet high in cadmium. The quail were fed 75 mg cadmium/kg for four weeks, which resulted in depressed growth, anemia and alteration in the essential elements in tissues. Vitamin C (1 percent) added to the diet produced a significant protective influence.

Dr. Chatterjee, et al., have reported on the dietary intake of metal ions and vitamin C metabolism. They have found that administration of any of the heavy metals—cadmium, lead or mercury—to rats reduces the levels of vitamin C in both the liver and kidneys. Lead was administered in these experiments at a dose of 10 mg/100 g body weight. Daily supplementation of the diet of these animals with vitamin C at a dose of 10 mg/100 g body weight raised vitamin C levels in tissues to above the control levels. Animal studies indicate that zinc and vitamin C may serve as antidotes for lead poisoning.

In any stress condition, whether it be infections, skin burns, post surgery cancer or even athletic training, the serum copper goes up and the zinc goes down. Competitive swimmers have a significantly higher serum copper level, according to G. Haralambe, et al. (1976).

Dr. Oleske has reported similar findings in asymptomatic lead-intoxicated children. He compared whole blood zinc and copper levels in a group of children with acute infection and an asymptomatic lead intoxication group with a control group admitted for elective surgery after minor trauma. The asymptomatic lead group was admitted for EDTA chelation therapy and had blood lead levels greater than 60 mcg percent. While the administration of zinc has been demonstrated to be beneficial in a number of stress states, no one has used zinc and vitamin C to reduce lead levels and symptoms.

Studies of the Brain Bio Center

This section surveys the psychiatric outpatient population of the Brain Bio Center and the use of vitamin C and zinc in treating lead-intoxicated individuals.

The blood lead levels of 1,113 outpatients were determined by the method of Hessel, and their serum copper levels were measured by atomic absorption spectroscopy of a trichloroacetic acid extract. Lead levels were determined for all subjects on the initial visit and for high lead patients on subsequent visits while they were on a regimen of vitamin C and zinc. Data were statistically analyzed by a paired t test.

The lead levels ranged from 3.8 to 53 mcg percent with a mean of 15.6 mcg percent; these levels agree with means reported in the literature for a general population. Six percent of the patients had lead levels above 25 mcg percent. The patients in this study were considered to have high lead values. Although levels below 40 mcg percent are generally considered to be non-toxic, attempts should be made to lower these levels, for every individual in a given population has unique susceptibilities and resistances. Symptoms of depression, anxiety, headache, sore joints and metallic taste were reported more frequently in the high lead group.

TABLE 18.2

Blood lead levels in adult male and female psychiatric outpatients on vitamin C and zinc therapy

	Male (n = 30) Mean ± S. D.		Female (n = 17) Mean ± S. D.	
Visit 1 (pretreatment)	24.6 ± 4.6 (mcg/%)		23.2 ± 2.8 (mcg/%)	
Visit 2	21.6 ± 5.9		18.2 ± 3.3	
Visit 3	18.8 ± 6.8		18.0 ± 5.1	
	t*	P	t	P
Visit 1 vs. 2	2.730	0.02	8.009	0.001
Visit 2 vs. 3	2.170	0.05	0.885	N.S.
Visit 1 vs. 3	5.082	0.001	4.539	0.001

* Paired t test.
N.S. = Not significant.
S.D. = Standard Deviation

Table 18.2 presents the results of zinc and vitamin C therapy on forty-seven adult patients. Blood lead levels were significantly reduced between the initial and subsequent visits. Oral daily dose levels are 2.0 gms vitamin C and 30 mg zinc as the gluconate A.M. and P.M. The difference in lead levels between the initial and third visit was significant at the 0.001 level when the data were analyzed with the paired t test. This means that this decrease would occur by chance only once in a thousand times. The effect of the treatment regimen was similar in both male and female patients. (My own blood lead level decreased with zinc and vitamin C as follows: 2–14–76 [22mcg percent], 5–14–76 [23 mcg percent], 11–13–76 [19 mcg percent], 1–3–77 [14 mcg percent], and 7–7–77 [10 mcg percent]. I plan to continue this simple regime to keep my lead and copper levels down.)

Children Respond to Zinc and Vitamin C

Children are more susceptible and have the unique symptom of hyperactivity when their lead and copper levels are high. Table 18.3 illustrates the findings of heavy metal burden in children with psychiatric problems. Not only lead but also copper may be a body and brain burden in these patients. We have shown previously that treatment with vitamin C and zinc will reduce the copper burden. In children, lead levels greater than their chronological age may be suspected to be the cause of hyperactivity, particularly in children with known lead exposure. A decrease in the heavy metal burden of copper and lead by treatment with vitamin C and zinc is followed by prompt clinical improvement. The remission may level off if the abnormal intake or exposure to lead and copper is not discovered and stopped. If the abnormal source is environmental, the patient should be moved to a lead-free environment; if the source of extra copper is in the drinking water, the patient should be given distilled water for drinking and for the preparation of foods.

Since the number of patients in this survey found to be suffering from lead intoxication was quite limited, we have recently instituted a study of twenty-two male lead workers with blood lead levels above 40 mcg percent. The efficacy of the proposed zinc and vitamin C therapy will be better validated with such a chronically exposed group.

TABLE 18.3

Heavy metal burden in hyperactive children

	Age	Lead mcg%	Copper mcg%	Serum Uric Acid
Male N = 19 % Elevated	10.7** ±2.2	18.2 ±5.0 100%	147 ±0.29 100%	4.1 1.7—6.7
Female N = 13 % Elevated	10.0 ±2.4	15.8 ±4.8 85%	134 ±0.16 100%	4.7 3.8—5.8

* Refers to a blood lead level greater than chronological age.
** Values expressed as mean ± standard deviation.

Lead Levels in Battery Workers

Storage batteries have a high lead content, and various lead salts are used in their manufacture. Lead pollution is apt to be high both in and around areas made dusty in the reclamation of lead from spent storage batteries.

Studies conducted in 1939 showed that lead-exposed workers treated with vitamin C experienced a decrease in blood lead, an increased number of red blood cells and hemoglobin content of blood, and a decrease in the number of stippled red blood cells. Even though a later 1943 study could not replicate these benefits, these investigators did establish that lead workers were more deficient in vitamin C than other workers.

If blood lead levels could be reduced for people who exhibited relatively low levels of lead, how effective would such treatment be for workers in lead-related industries who suffer exposure to high levels of lead all day year after year? It would be a great boon to the industry if workers could be protected against accumulating toxic levels of lead by the use of simple nutrients such as vitamin C and zinc.

Forty men from a local battery plant, whose ages ranged from twenty-eight to sixty years and who were

Figure 18.1

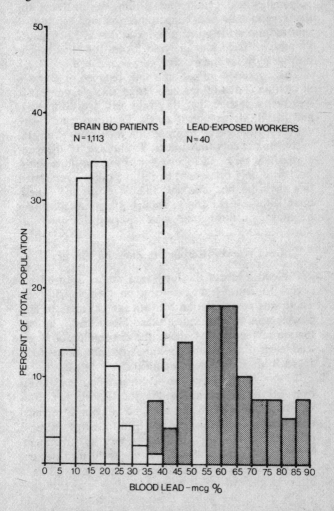

employed at the plant for four to thirty-four years, visited our laboratories in the early spring of 1976. Samples were taken for determinations in whole blood of lead, copper, erythrocyte protoporphyrin, histamine, polyamines and glutathione. Serum was analyzed for the trace metals, zinc, copper and iron, and serum was sent to an outside laboratory for a SMAC 22 diagnostic profile. Urine was analyzed for fat-soluble Ehrlich-positive pyrroles and for zinc, copper and lead.

The workers were put on a daily regimen of 2 grams of vitamin C and 60 mg zinc (from zinc gluconate). It was recommended that they take half the dose A.M. and half P.M. with their meals. Of the original forty workers, twenty-five returned for follow-up after six, twelve and twenty-four weeks. Twenty-two of them reported that they had followed the program quite faithfully with only occasional lapses; the other three stated that they did not take any vitamin C or zinc. These three, although not a large enough sample to constitute a significant control group, were observed closely.

Lead Workers Respond to Zinc and Vitamin C

The blood levels of the forty lead workers ranged between 36 and 89 mcg percent on their initial visit. There was no correlation between age or length of employment in the lead industry and blood lead. The histogram in Figure 18.1 shows the distribution of blood lead levels of these subjects compared with those of the 1,113 Brain Bio Center outpatients.

Twelve of the forty subjects had blood lead levels over 60 mcg percent on the initial visit but after twenty-four weeks on the zinc and vitamin C regimen only four still had this lead level. In fact, this decrease occurred within the first six weeks of treatment. Whereas only two subjects had under 40 mcg percent lead on the initial visit, this figure increased to six men after six and twelve weeks and to eight at twenty-four weeks. Using the paired t test, the decrease in blood lead from a mean level of 61.6 ± 14.9 to 46.9 ± 14.9

after twenty-four weeks of treatment was highly significant ($p < 0.001$).

Serum zinc levels increased in the first six weeks of therapy from 112.6 to 143.0, demonstrating the initial rise we normally see in patients beginning zinc supplementation, and then fell back characteristically to normal levels by twenty-four weeks. There was no significant correlation between initial serum zinc and blood lead levels, nor between the extent of rise in zinc and the fall in lead.

The serum copper was somewhat higher for the lead workers (114.3 ± 13.7) versus the controls (107 ± 23.7), and there was a significant drop ($p < 0.01$) during the period of treatment to 103.4 ± 19.1. Whole blood copper also dropped significantly. There was no essential difference in serum iron levels between the lead workers and the controls, nor any change with treatment.

The lead workers showed characteristic disturbances in all the blood cell tests. The mean hemoglobin level was $13.4 \pm .78$ at the pretreatment level versus 15.3 ± 1.2 for the 100 male controls, lower even than the mean of 13.9 for a control group of females. The mean hemoglobin increased to 14.3 ± 1.6 ($p < 0.01$) after twenty-four weeks of treatment. There was no significant correlation between initial hemoglobin levels and initial blood lead levels. The mean red blood cell protoporphyrin was high (149.8 ± 132.4 mcg percent RBC) and remained elevated throughout the course of treatment. However, twenty-four weeks may be too short a period to note improvement in blood cells due to their long life span (120 days). Furthermore, we were observing workers during a period when they were continually exposed to lead.

Other biochemical findings were that the lead workers had high serum uric acid levels—levels that were related to job location (those working in areas with the highest lead exposure had the highest uric acid levels). We also found blood spermine levels to be elevated.

We believe that the decrease in blood lead levels

that occurred during the twenty-four week period during which the twenty-two lead workers were taking zinc and vitamin C was striking inasmuch as the men were simultaneously on the job and were therefore constantly exposed to lead (except for a two-week period, the eighteenth to twentieth week of study when the entire plant was closed for vacation). The three men not taking treatment showed no significant change in blood lead levels.

Questions for the Future

Our study was a pilot study and as such leaves many questions unanswered. We do not know, for example, if the zinc and vitamin C regimen is therapeutic or prophylactic, or both. Is the old lead, the accumulation of years in the body tissues and bone where some 90 percent of the body's burden is stored, being mobilized and removed from the body? Or is the vitamin regimen preventing the absorption of new lead? If the latter, men newly entering the lead industry may be protected against lead poisoning by taking zinc and vitamin C.

It has been reported that the blood lead levels of twenty men entering employment in the lead industry climbed to a mean level of 60 mcg percent (with a range of 50 to 80 mcg percent) within three weeks and stayed there for the duration of the twelve week study. This is the same mean and range as that for the group working with lead for four to thirty-four years. A most interesting study would be to screen men entering the lead industry for the first time. Their blood lead levels and perhaps other physiological measurements that change with lead exposure would be monitored and compared with those of a similiar group of men, matched by age and job location, who would be on a daily regimen of zinc and vitamin C. Such an investigation would require only several weeks if only the blood lead levels were studied, and it could resolve whether our recommended treatment is an effective preventive of lead poisoning.

Another simple study that might indicate whether

the zinc and vitamin C regimen is reducing body stores of lead rather than acting simply as a preventive against entry of new lead would be to monitor men leaving a lead-using industry. Would a group on vitamin C and zinc have an accelerated decrease in blood lead levels or an accelerated improvement in other lead-related biochemical parameters as compared with untreated retirees?

Even though some questions do remain unanswered, we believe the results of our study warrant the use of our vitamin program by lead-exposed workers, and we are eager to see a lead-using industry activate our nutrient program.

Significance of Lead Reduction by Zinc and Vitamin C

From a number of points of view, the therapy proposed may be advantageous. For example, the current treatment of lead poisoning involves chelation therapy with agents such as EDTA or penicillamine, both of which are much more hazardous than zinc and vitamin C. Moreover, a number of studies have shown kidney damage due to prolonged or reckless use of Ca EDTA, which has been used as a prophylactic measure in a number of instances with lead-exposed workers. This practice is deplorable in that environmental conditions for the exposure are not alleviated and the worker may be harmed by the possible toxic effects of the medication. Our nutrient therapy is simple, cheap and relatively free of side-effects.

Children Present Special Problems

The problem of lead exposure in children deserves some further comment since it is well established that lead poisoning in children is quite different from that observed in adults. In adults, the lead exposure is generally connected with a known dangerous occupation; in children exposure is often due to consumption of foreign particles such as paint chips or inhalation as a result of living near a super-highway.

It appears that children absorb lead more easily and retain it to a greater extent than adults. In contrast to the adult where lead is stored primarily in bone, in children large amounts of lead remain in the soft tissues. The results of this study suggest that most children with psychiatric problems should first be checked for both lead and copper poisoning.

The problem of a high lead burden in children has been discussed extensively by Drs. Bryce-Smith and Waldren. In children who are clinically asymptomatic of food poisoning and whose lead levels are not markedly above 40 mcg percent, they have found a broad range of psychological impairment. In addition, hyperactive children with blood lead levels of the order of 25 mcg percent have shown great improvement when treated with penicillamine or calcium-EDTA. For our part, we believe that in hyperactive children lead levels of 15 to 25 mcg percent may be suspect, and even lead levels above the actual age of the patient when the serum uric acid is high.

In summary, blood levels on over 1,000 psychiatric outpatients indicate that lead exposure may cause psychiatric symptoms in a definite percentage, particularly in hyperactive children. A zinc and ascorbic acid dietary supplementation results in a decrease in their blood lead and copper levels.

Acknowledgment

The author is indebted to Arthur Sohler, Ph.D., and Rhoda Papaioannou, M.S., for the collaborative lead findings in Brain Bio Center patients.

TABLE 18.4

Toxic effects of lead in man

Gastro-intestinal

| Constipation | Nausea | Colic |
| Discolored gums | Diarrhea | Loss of appetite |

Muscles and joints

| Easy fatigue | Muscle weakness and cramps | Bone and joint atrophy |
| Gout | Rheumatoid arthritis | Lead line on X ray |

Brain and nerves

Clumsiness	Restlessness	Vertigo
Insomnia	Mental retardation	Loss of coordination
Headache	Confusion	Irritability
Paralysis	Tremors	Emotional instability

Blood

| Anemia | Low hemoglobin | Stippled red cells |

TABLE 18.5

Multiple sources of lead contamination in man

Urban atmophere	Printing	Lead pipes
Gasoline additives	Wines	Construction materials
Paints and enamels	Insecticides	Cigarette smoke
Ceramic glazes	Hair coloring	Plaster
Solder	Putty	Glass
Plating	Batteries	Ammunition—target practice
Crayons	Foundries	Machine shops
Newsprint	Comics	Industry environments
Hobbies	Leaded glass	Lead reclamation
Catalogs	Hearth dust	Lead soldiers
Road dust	Bone meal?	Vegetables from roadside gardens

References

Allen, B. R.; Moore, M. R. and Hunter, J. A. A. Lead and the skin. *British Journal of Dermatology* 92:715, 1975.

Altman, L. K. Retardation link to lead is found. Study of Scottish children reports on contamination of drinking water. *The New York Times,* 31 March 1975.

Ammerman, C. B.; Miller, S. M.; Fick, K. R. and Hansard, S. L. Contaminating elements in mineral supplements and their potential toxicity. A review. *Journal of Animal Science* 44(3):485, 1977.

Baloh, R.; Sturm, R.; Green, B. and Gleser, G. Neuropsychological effects of chronic asymptomatic increased lead absorption. A controlled study. *Archives of Neurology* 32:326–330, May 1975.

Beattie, A. D. Diagnostic and therapeutic uses of D-penicillamine in lead poisoning. *Postgraduate Medical Journal,* August Suppl. 1974, pp. 17–20.

Bronson, G. Study shows children of lead workers are susceptible to lead-dust poisoning. *Wall Street Journal,* 3 February 1977.

Chamberlain, A. C.; Heard, M. J.; Stott, A. N. B.; Clough, W. S.; Newton, D. and Wells, A. C. Uptake of inhaled lead from motor exhaust. *Postgraduate Medical Journal* 51:790–794, November 1975.

Crosby, W. H. Lead-contaminated health food. Association with lead poisoning and leukemia. *JAMA* 237(24):2627–2629, 13 June 1977.

David, O.; Hoffman, S.; Sverd, J.; Clark, J. and Voeller, K. Lead and hyperactivity. Behavioral response to chelation: a pilot study. *American Journal of Psychiatry* 133(10):1155–1158, October 1976.

David, O.; McGann, B.; Hoffman, S.; Sverd, J. and Clark, J. Low lead levels and mental retardation. *The Lancet,* 25 December 1976, pp. 1376–1379.

Does lead make children hyperactive? *Nutrition Reviews* 31(3):88–90, March 1973.

Fischbein, A. and Lilis, R. Bystanders at risk of lead absorption. *The Lancet*, 26 March 1977.

Hammond, P. B. Exposure of humans to lead. *Annual Reviews Pharmacology Toxicology* 17:197–214, 1977.

High lead content: a problem of old-fashioned soldered cans. *Consumer Reports*, February 1976.

Hussey, H. H. Lead poisoning and fecundity in men. *JAMA* (Editorial) 233:7, 18 August 1975.

Hyatt, J. C. New lead-disease data spur U.S. to ask smelters to tighten controls on exposure. *Wall Street Journal*, 23 February 1976.

Jugo, S.; Maljkovic, T. and Kostial, K. Influence of chelating agents on the gastrointestinal absorption of lead. *Toxicology and Applied Pharmacology* 34:259–263, 1975.

Kopito, L. E. and Schwachman, H. Lead in human scalp hair, some factors affecting its variability. *Journal of Investigative Dermatology* 64:342–348, 1975.

Landrigan, P. J. and Baker, E. L. Child health and environmental lead. *British Medical Journal* 836, 26 March 1977.

Landrigan, P. J.; Baloh, R. W.; Barthel, W. F.; Whitworth, R. H.; Staehling, N. W. and Rosenblum, B. F. Neuropsychological dysfunction in children with chronic low-level lead absorption. *The Lancet*, March 1975.

Lead and mental retardation. *Science News* 107:222, 1976.

Levander, O. A. Nutritional factors in relation to heavy metal toxicants. *Fed. Proc.* 36(5):1683–1687, April 1977.

Lublin, J. S. Health foods blamed in illness physicians couldn't diagnose—actress discovers big doses of a calcium supplement gave her lead poisoning. *Wall Street Journal*, 14 June 1977.

Mitchell, D. G. Increased lead absorption: paint is not the only problem. *Pediatrics* 53:2, February 1974.

Morgan, J. M. Chelation therapy in lead nephropathy. *Southern Medical Journal* 68(8):1001–1006, August 1975.

Morrison, J. H.; Olton, D. S.; Goldberg, A. M. and Silbergeld, E. K. Alterations in consummatory behavior of mice produced by dietary exposure to inorganic lead. *Developmental Psychobiology* 8(5):389–396, 1975.

Ng, R. Lead poisoning from lead-soldered electric kettles. *CMA Journal* 116:508–512, 5 March 1977.

Niklowitz, W. J. Neurofibrillary changes after acute experimental lead poisoning. *Neurology* 25(10):927–934, October 1975.

Niklowitz, W. J. and Mandybur, T. I. Neurofibrillary changes following childhood lead encephalopathy. *Journal of Neuropathology and Experimental Neurology* 34(5):445–455, September 1975.

Oleske, J. M.; Valentine, J. L. and Minnefor, A. B. The effects of acute infection of blood lead, copper, and zinc levels in children. *Health Laboratory Science* 12(3):230–233, July 1975.

Orfanos, C. E. and Künzig, M. Chronische Bleiintoxikation: Bleigicht mit Riesentophi an der Haut, Nephropathie und Porphyrinopathie. *Der Hautarzt* 26:581–584, 1975.

Püschel, S. M. Bleiintoxikation im Kindesalter: Eine "silent Epidemic" in den Slums der Vereinigten Staaten. *Klin Pädiat.* 187:395–400, 1975.

Rom, W. N. Effects of lead on the female and reproduction: a review. *Mount Sinai Journal of Medicine* 43(5):542–551, September/October 1976.

Sauerhoff, M. W. and Michaelson, I. A. Hyperactivity and brain catecholamines in lead-exposed developing rats. *Science* 182:1022–1024, 7 December 1973.

Senility and lead. *BioMedicine* 313, 15 November 1975.

Silbergeld, E. K. and Goldberg, A. M. Lead-induced behavioral dysfunction: an animal model of hyperactivity. *Experimental Neurology* 42:146–157, 1974.

Spivey-Fox, M. R. Protective effects of ascorbic acid against toxicity of heavy metals. *Annals of the New York Academy of Sciences* 258:144–149, 1975.

Wedeen, R. P.; Maesaka, J. K.; Weiner, B.; Lipat, G. A.; Lyons, M. M.; Vitale, L. F. and Joselow, M. M. Occupational lead nephropathy. *American Journal of Medicine* 59:630–641, November 1975.

White, D. J. Histochemical and histological effects of lead on the liver and kidney of the dog. *British Journal of Experimental Pathology* 58:101–112, 1977.

Zetterlund, B.; Winberg, J.; Lundgren, W. and Johansson, G. Lead in umbilical cord blood correlated with the blood lead of the mother in areas with low, medium or high atmospheric pollution. *Acta Paediatr. Scand.* 66:169–175, 1977.

Copper:
The Fourth
Heavy-Metal Intoxicant

Our Body Burden of Copper

As we have seen, the heavy metals lead, mercury and cadmium are poisons which slowly accumulate with age as a body burden, much as barnacles accumulate on a ship at sea. This body burden can shorten life by the production of hardening of the arteries, high blood pressure, kidney disease, psychosis, early senility and numerous other diseases of aging. We now have sufficient evidence to incriminate a fourth metal, copper, as a culpable heavy metal.

Copper Is Too Much with Us

Copper is essential in small amounts to form hemoglobin. This discovery was made by Dr. E. B. Hart of the University of Wisconsin in 1928, but work on the intimate metabolism of copper is proceeding slowly. Copper can be found in all iron salts and in many foods, so that adult man can be considered safe from copper deficiency. Dr. Gubler, in an excellent review published in 1956, states, "It is doubtful that an unquestioned case of copper deficiency has been reported in man. It is also extremely unlikely that copper deficiency could occur in man even on suboptimal diets." We have determined serum copper in more than seventeen hundred patients and have not found a single case of copper deficiency. In our present environment, we are satiated with copper, so that only premature infants and patients on parenteral (intravenous) feedings have shown copper deficiency. Anyone who eats and drinks gets copper!

The body of an adult contains 125 mg of copper; the liver, via the bile, is the main route of excretion of excess copper. The liver has the highest copper content, the brain is second, and other organs and tissues contain much less. Fetal liver at term contains approximately seven times as much copper as adult liver. Five to fifteen years are needed to bring the level of copper down to the adult level. Since copper is a stimulant to the brain, this excess copper may be a factor in the hyperactivity in children which ameliorates with age and slow elimination of the copper burden. This excess of copper in the young is also evident in sheep and cows. Lambs' and calves' livers are much higher in copper than are the livers from the full-grown animals.

Postpartum Psychosis

We quote as follows from R. Gooch (1820):

> It is well known that some women, who are perfectly sane at all other times, become deranged after delivery, and that this form of the disease is called puerperal insanity. My situation gives me more than the common opportunities of seeing it and, though I am unable to make any important additions to our knowledge of the subject, I have witnessed some things which seem to me to deserve attention: these I will venture to describe, together with what I have observed about the causes, progress, and treatment of this distressing malady.
>
> The most common time for the disease to begin is a few days, or a few weeks, after delivery; sometimes it happens after several months, during nursing, or soon after weaning.
>
> The approach of the disease is announced by symptoms which excite little apprehension because they so often occur without any such termination; the

pulse is quick without any manifest cause, the nights are restless, and the temper is sharp; soon, however, there is an indescribable hurry, and peculiarity of manner, which a watchful and experienced observer, and those accustomed to the patient will notice; her conduct and language become wild and incoherent; and at length she becomes decidedly maniacal; it is fortunate if she does not attempt her life before the nature of the malady is discovered.

Copper, and particularly ceruloplasmin (a copper-containing protein) is elevated by estrogens; therefore, the levels of copper and ceruloplasmin rise progressively during pregnancy. Serum copper is approximately 115 mcg percent at conception, and reaches a mean of 260 mcg percent at term. After delivery, a period of two to three months is required before the original serum copper level is reached. This high postpartum copper level may be a factor in causing postpartum depression and psychosis; more data are needed in this area. One must also discover the differences in copper metabolism when the pregnant schizophrenic patient carries a male or female child. We know that the incidence of postpartum psychosis is much greater after the birth of a male child. If the estrogen level alone were the cause, one would expect the reverse.

According to Ylastalo and Reinila, the exaggerated rise in serum copper may be a factor in toxemia of pregnancy (preeclampsia level, 287 v. 258 for normals) and in hepatosis (inflammation and enlargement of the liver) or pregnancy (serum copper, 342 mcg percent). Pfeiffer and Iliev have found that the oral contraceptive, with its potent estrogen, raises copper in schizophrenics to a level higher than that of the ninth month of pregnancy. This rise produces activation of their psychoses which may last for several weeks after stopping the pill. The remission of the psychosis corresponds to the slow decline of accumulated copper in the blood and tissues.

Dietary Copper

Copper is an essential element for supporting life, but, in excess, copper can be toxic. Environmental factors can cause copper and iron overloading. The foods we eat and the water we drink affect our delicate balance, depending on the environment and the material of the water piping. The average adult ingests 3 to 5 mg per day. Since the actual adult need is closer to 2 mg per day, an accumulation may occur.

From a biochemical point of view, surplus dietary copper can cause severe physical and mental illness. Although additional copper sulfate may promote growth in various animals, it would be prudent to consider the effect that this dietary supplement might have on those people eating the meat products. Even those who refrain from eating meat may be subject to copper intoxication; soybeans contain a significant amount of copper. Research is now under way on growing soybeans with extra zinc and manganese so that individuals relying on this product for their intake of protein will not be nutritionally deficient or too high in any one trace element.

Deficiency of Zinc Accentuates Copper Excess

Food-processing techniques deprive foods of many nutrients. Wheat, for example, has twenty-three nutrients crushed, ground and squeezed out of it during processing. This processing is designed to reduce trace metal content since such removal prolongs the shelf life. During the freezing process, fresh green vegetables are "blanched with sequestrants" to produce a bright green color when cooked. However, the zinc and manganese content is reduced to 20 percent of the normal range! A European diet provides more zinc and manganese than the American diet. Europeans consume homemade soups and fresh vegetables and drink wines, while Americans seem to favor frozen foods, ice cream, soft drinks and artificial fruit juices. Because the food we eat and the water we drink influence our physical and mental health, we should investigate the possibility that many of the devices used to promote growth in plants and animals and to process our foods may be detrimental to our own minds and bodies.

Copper in the Water We Use

Critical attention is now focused on certain elements in man's drinking water that may, in toxic quantities, cause severe physiological and mental illnesses or death. Pfeiffer and Iliev have shown that in some suburban homes, individual water systems where the well water is usually acid can produce copper intoxication. As an example of the copper in drinking water, look at these data from a suburban home in Peapack, New Jersey. The well water has 0.03 ppm of copper, the upper bath has 0.32 ppm and an outside faucet has 1.62 ppm. In the house, only the upper bathroom tap has drinkable water by United States Public Health Service (USPHS) standards (maximum 1 ppm).

TABLE 19.1

Typical copper content of home waters*
Resident water in Peapack, N.J., 22 June 1974

	Copper content
Well	0.03 ppm
Upstairs bath	0.32 ppm
Kitchen—Calgon charcoal filter	1.24 ppm
Outside faucet	1.62 ppm

* The dripping faucets of this home were noted for producing blue deposits on the porcelain. A brass filter containing charcoal was installed in the kitchen. This did not correct the basic fault, namely acid well water which leaches copper from the plumbing and even from the brass of the filter. Some outside, unused faucets can have copper levels of 50 ppm.

A recent report from Australia confirms the gravity of this finding. A new well was bored on an Australian farm and new copper plumbing was installed, complete with a copper hot-water tank. The mother was four months pregnant when the family moved to the farm. At birth, the male infant was not breast fed but rather bottle fed, with water from the tap being used to make the infant's formula. The child died at fourteen months of age with all the symptoms and findings of chronic copper intoxication.

Upon examination the well water had an acid pH of 3.8 to 4.8 (normal 7.0) and a copper content as high as 970 mcg percent. (The upper limit for drinking water set by the USPHS is 100 mcg percent.) The family was tested and all showed normal copper except the mother who, when given penicillamine (a chelating agent) excreted large amounts of copper. This suggests that copper excess could have started in utero. This death is the first to be reported from copper in the drinking water, but many previous deaths have been reported from copper poisoning.

Serum zinc deficiency and serum copper excess have become evident only since the change from galvanized waterpipes to copper plumbing. Before copper plumbing, man obtained his needed supply of zinc by drinking water which had coursed through zinc-lined (galvanized) pipes. As a result of the installation of copper plumbing in conjunction with the slight acidity of most drinkable water, we are getting an excess of copper which may be antagonizing the zinc we obtain from food. This is most likely when water is pumped from shale or loam. In some areas of New Jersey, well water will produce pin holes in copper piping in ten years' time. The copper goes into the drinking water! (See Table 19.2)

In subacute poisoning of rats with copper, Lal et al. have found great increases in liver copper and some deaths. The activity of a zinc-containing enzyme, lactic acid dehydrogenase, was decreased, as was that of the enzyme which destroys amines in the brain when they are no longer needed. Brain copper increased 36 percent in a six-week period, and the turnover of serotonin was apparently reduced. The adrenal glands markedly increased in weight—an index of stress.

TABLE 19.2

Copper content of some drinking waters in the eastern United States[a]

Location	Water source	Dwelling	Copper content (ppm)[b]
New York City	River	Apartment	0.07
Long Island	Well	Cottage	0.03
Cleveland	Lake	Motel	0.06
Boston	Well	House	0.12[c]
Greenwich, Conn.	Well	House	0.35[c]
Greenwich	Well	House	0.37[c]
Wilton, Conn.	Well	House	1.60[c]
Wilton	Well	House	1.34[c]
Wilton	Well	House	0.68[c]
Wilton	Well	House	0.36[c]
Wilton	Well	House	0.40[c]
Wilton	Well	House	0.18[c]
New Canaan, Conn.	Well	House	0.85[c]
Redding, Conn.	Well	House	4.20[c]
Belle Mead, N.J.	Well	Clinic	0.12
Bernardsville, N.J.	Well	House	0.54[c]
Princeton, N.J.	Well	House	0.05
Princeton	Well	House	0.11
Princeton	Well	House	0.04
Princeton	Well	House	0.06[c]
Milwood, N.J.	Well	House	0.09
Trenton, N.J.	Well	House	5.60[c]
Stamford, Conn.	Well	House	5.20[c]
Boston	Well	House	0.64[c]
Atlantic City, N.J.	River	House	0.01[c]
Dayton, Ohio	Well	House	0.56[c]
Washington, D.C.	River	Hotel	0.01

Excess copper in the body may play a role in certain diseases. Mildred Seelig, in 1973, researched the role of the copper-molybdenum interaction in certain iron-deficiency anemias and has postulated that a high copper-molybdenum ratio in the American diet may contribute to iron-deficiency anemias and possibly cause iron-storage diseases. There is evidence that elevated serum copper levels decrease iron during pregnancy and also result in a conditioned molybdenum deficiency. According to Butt et al., the trace-metal pattern of iron-storage diseases suggests a relationship of iron, molybdenum, lead and possibly copper to the cause of these diseases. Several anemias that do not respond to iron therapy have been found to be associated with high copper levels.

Copper and Cadmium in Plated Containers

All soluble salts of copper and cadmium are strong emetics (produce vomiting) when taken in sufficient dosage. Zinc and nickel sulfates are milder emetics, in that a larger dose is needed to produce vomiting. This means that epidemics of nausea and vomiting can occur when acid syrups such as cola or lemon drinks are stored in automatic dispensing machines. Since the effect is dose-/body-weight related, the young child who attends the Saturday afternoon matinee may have serious nausea and vomiting if he happens to get the first drink of the day from the soft-drink dispenser. Acid syrup, standing in contact with the tubes and valves overnight, may accumulate a dose of cadmium

---

a All waters were collected in plastic containers and were acidified with copper-free HCL prior to testing. The sample was the first collection of water in the morning.

b The USPHS has ruled that water containing more than 1.0 ppm of copper is unfit to drink. In earlier generations with lead plumbing, grandfather, who drank the first cup out of the faucet in the morning, often got lead poisoning. It is now possible in some suburban homes for grandfather or others to get copper poisoning.

c Indicates a family in which at least one member has psychiatric problems.

and copper which is toxic in a 50-pound child. The adult male might only get nausea, while the child may have repeated vomiting. In such cases, both child and adult add to their body burden of copper and cadmium.

We first witnessed this phenomenon in the U.S. Navy, where our duty included the review of all courts-martial proceedings. We had such gems as, "U.S. Navy v John Doe, Seaman First Class, who did urinate on the deck of the Cruiser Tuscaloosa *while the nation was at war.*" But, more seriously, we had submarines which were forced to abort their Pacific cruises because of epidemic nausea and vomiting. Those who could work manned their posts while the sub went back to Pearl Harbor without firing a single torpedo—hence the court-martial inquiry.

After eliminating the possibility that the cause was arsenic and antimony poisoning from contaminated plates of the storage batteries, we finally found the root of the problem in an ice cream soda fountain that had recently been installed aboard these submarines. In wartime, because nickel was scarce, the syrup containers were *cadmium* plated. The soda fountain was open only once a week, so any acid syrups accumulated great amounts of cadmium from the six days' exposure to the surface. Men who preferred chocolate did not get sick, but the favorite flavor was raspberry (very acid) and all who preferred raspberry sundaes got deathly sick, with nausea and vomiting, from the cadmium content. All epidemics stopped when plastic containers were substituted for the cadmium-plated containers.

The insidious nature of heavy-metal poisoning should alert the consumer, the physician and the epidemiologist to all risk factors of modern life if poisoning is to be restrained to a reasonable level.

Excess Copper as a Possible Cause of Autism

The changes in copper and iron storage which occur during pregnancy, suckling and infancy were reviewed by Linder and Munro in 1973. We know that during the suckling period breast milk is deficient in copper and iron; the amount of excess copper and iron stored in the infant's liver should therefore decrease in the first six months of life. At this time, the liver produces the normal copper protein, ceruloplasmin, which stores copper in the blood serum and prevents excess absorption. Similarly, ferritin, the iron-containing protein, is made. Any abnormality which results in inadequate ceruloplasmin or ferritin could allow excess copper or iron to be absorbed, which would affect the brain. Both of these metals are stimulants to the brain and might produce hyperactivity or autism, with development into adulthood being slow or failing to take place normally. Nothing in the fetal development process protects against excess copper and iron. An alternative hypothesis is that heavy metals such as lead and mercury could interfere with the synthesis of ceruloplasmin or ferritin. This theory is worthy of testing, and can be tested by the usual laboratory methods in autistic children.

Tap Water, Blood and Dementia

The use of tap water as a dialysis substance has probably resulted in many unexpected deaths. "Dementia dialytica" was first described in 1964 by Peterson and Swanson. Patients had psychiatric changes which ranged from stuttering to aphasia (loss or impairment of the ability to use words as symbols of ideas) to unreality and cardiac standstill—with many symptoms in between (see Table 19.3)! Lindner et al. have found that patients subjected to dialysis can develop fulminating arteriosclerosis which could have been caused by cadmium, copper or a great deficiency of zinc. The anemias of pregnancy, rheumatoid arthritis and infection show high levels of ceruloplasmin. Wilson's disease has been associated with the high copper/molybdenum ratio, especially in the liver.

TABLE 19.3

"Dementia dialytica": clinical mystery or diagnostic dichotomy?

Psychiatric, neurological, and medical symptoms of hemodialysis patients using tap water

Psychiatric diagnosis since 1964 (Peterson and Swanson) termed "Dementia dialytica"	*Medical diagnosis since 1969 (Matter, et al.) Tap-water dialysis increases serum copper*

Neurological symptoms	*Medical symptoms*
Speech disorder, slow articulation	Hemolytic anemia, hematuria (Ivanovich, et al. 1969)
Stuttering, aphasia, headaches	Lowered hematocrit with right (liver) or left (spleen) upper quadrant pain (Manzler and Schreiner, 1970)
EEG: Slow waves with delta waves and spikes. (Alfrey, et al. 1972)	
Myoclonus, convulsions	Green plasma
Hypertension, restlessness	Nausea, vomiting
Increased heart rate and irregularities	Yellow, watery diarrhea
Cardiac standstill	Weakness, syncope

Psychiatric symptoms	*Psychiatric symptoms*
Inability to concentrate	Unreality
Impaired memory	Depression

Personality changes	Psychosis
Psychotic behavior	
"Disequilibrium syndrome" (unknown changes in vasoactive amines) *Journal of the American Medical Association* **224:1578 (1973)**; Ibid **226:190 (1973)**	*Pathological symptoms*
	Increased tin in brain at autopsy

Psychiatric Theories (*Halper, 1971*)	*Medical theories*
Dependency increases aggressive feelings (dependency on public finances) **Defenses all brittle** **Stress: anxiety, depression, paranoia and suicidal tendencies** **Denial of aspects of reality** **Decreased sex activity**	**Heavy metal intoxication** **Copper intoxication** **(Mahler,** et al., **1971)**

Copper in the tap water may turn the blood plasma green since copper accumulates preferentially in plasma. Symptoms have been described since 1964, but only in 1969 was the syndrome correlated with excess copper or other heavy metals such as tin. In some instances, according to Barbour et al., copper tubing or copperized plastic was involved. Excess copper would appear to be the most likely cause since some schizophrenics improve when their excess copper is removed. Cross-references between the two columns are so rare as to suggest a dichotomy of diagnosis and thinking.

When the quantity of copper-containing protein, ceruloplasmin, is adequate in the blood, it inhibits the intestinal absorption of copper. But if, as is the case in Wilson's disease, the serum contains an insufficient amount of ceruloplasmin, copper is absorbed in excess and diffuses into the tissues, and may accumulate in high levels in the brain and liver, producing severe mental illness and death. Fortunately, Wilson's disease is rare; in more than seventeen hundred psychiatric patients studied for copper levels, we have not found a single case of Wilson's disease.

Copper and Heart Attacks

Cases of myocardial infarction in people under forty are increasing in the United States, which is already the world leader in this disease. The recent studies of Dr. Oscar Roth of the Yale University School of Medicine reveal that the rate is twenty-seven times higher in men than in women, but that women on oral contraceptive medication may have a much greater risk. He has observed five tragic cases of myocardial infarction in women on the pill. Serum copper is high with use of the birth control pill, and the copper level of the heart is higher than normal in those dying from heart attacks. Copper is also high in patients with high blood pressure and in those who smoke. We therefore postulate that the smoking woman, on oral contraceptives, who lives in suburbia where well water is used and is at the same time under stress (which dissipates zinc) and who has borderline zinc deficiency may have the greatest susceptibility to early heart attacks or strokes.

Copper and One Type of Schizophrenia

Thus far, excessive copper levels have been associated with our bodies' disorders, but in recent studies of the various schizophrenias, Pfeiffer et al. have postulated that excessive copper and iron and/or zinc and manganese deficiency are primary factors in one type of schizophrenia, namely histapenia. Histaminase is a copper-containing enzyme, and both histaminase and ceruloplasm can destroy histamine. Therefore, patients with high serum copper and ceruloplasm have low levels of blood histamine. Histapenic schizophrenia responds to treatment which rids the body of copper and builds up blood and tissue histamine.

Our studies indicate that a possible factor in some of the schizophrenias is a combined deficiency of zinc and manganese with a relative increase in iron and copper, or both—the copper possibly originating from copper plumbing. The urinary copper excretion in schizophrenics is consistently less than in "normal" patients; zinc plus manganese in dietary doses is effective in increasing copper elimination and reducing copper to normal levels. Further research is needed to determine the exact roles of these elements in vascular and brain chemistry. If, in fact, zinc deficiency and copper excess are crucial factors in causation of one of the schizophrenias, then more evidence is needed on the exact causes of these imbalances, so that treatment can be facilitated and prevention provided.

The clinical syndromes (other than Wilson's disease) wherein elevated serum or tissue copper may be an important factor are paranoid and hallucinatory schizophrenia, hypertension, stuttering, autism, childhood hyperactivity, preeclampsia, premenstrual tensions, psychiatric depression, insomnia, senility, and the possibly functional hypoglycemia. Postpartum psychosis and the newborn infant's burden of copper have been described.

How to Lower Our Copper Burden

We have said that copper is essential for life, that excess copper accumulated in the body can be dangerous to good health, and that the general knowledge that the metals lead and mercury can cause insanity has now been extended to copper. We must now ask, how does one rid the body of its burden of excess copper?

It has long been held that a well-balanced diet is all that is needed. It is true that a perfectly balanced diet is so replete in all essential minerals that the zinc, manganese and molybdenum content would antagonize copper and prevent any accumulation. However, soil, fertilizers, foods and people are seldom tested for anything other than heavy metals and iron. On the basis of hemoglobin determinations, the teen-ager and the young adult have been labeled iron deficient. We know, however, that pyridoxine (B-6) and zinc are also involved in hemoglobin synthesis. Our deficient soils lower the levels of trace elements in our plants. Food processors continue to remove 90 percent of the zinc, manganese, molybdenum and pyridoxine from wheat grain, while enriching white flour with more iron) patients. The present white flour should be called in a higher incidence of gray-skinned siderotic (high-iron) patients. The present white flour should be called "tinkered ersatz" rather than "enriched." Additional tinkering should be in the direction of restoring zinc, manganese and magnesium content to the original level found in the wheat grain.

TABLE 19.4

Selected foodstuffs with appreciable amounts of copper

mg/100gm

Meats

beef liver	2.80
beef heart	.29
calf liver	7.90
duck liver	4.87
lamb liver	5.60
pork liver	1.14
veal chops	.25
pork chops	.31
lamb chops	.24
mutton, leg	.24
chicken breast	.18
chicken wing	.22
bacon	.52

Seafood

crab, canned	1.52
lobster	1.69
oysters	17.14
shrimp, fresh	.60
tuna, fresh	.50

Dairy Products

cream	.11
eggs, fresh	.10
milk, condensed	.22

Nuts and Seeds

brazil nuts	1.53
filberts	1.23
peanuts	.62
pecans	1.14
walnuts	1.39
sesame seeds	1.59
sunflower seeds	1.77
pistachio nuts	1.12

Spices

curry powder	1.07
pepper, black	.58
salt	.44

Dried Fruits

apricots	.35
dates	.22
figs	.28
prunes	.28
raisins	.25

Vegetables

avocados	.39
kidney beans	.84
lima beans	.73
navy beans	.85
mushrooms	1.00
peas	.22
soybeans	1.17
yams	.22

Cereals

bran flakes	.61
Cheerios	.44
Puffed Rice	.39
Rice Krispies	.30
wheat flakes	.44

Breads

brown	.28
rye	.23
wheat	.24
white	.23

Grains

wheat bran	1.45
wheat germ	2.39
corn, white	.24
corn germ	1.01
rice	.28

Sweets

sugar wafers	.84
chocolate (bitter)	2.67
chocolate (sweet)	1.04

jam, all kinds	.31	ground coffee	1.26
molasses	1.42	tea, bag	4.80
licorice	.39	tea, instant dry	1.10
		Instant Breakfast (Carnation) dry	.50
Condiments		Instant Breakfast (PET) dry	6.25
mustard	.40		
olives	.34		
sweet relish	.50	*Miscellaneous*	
catsup	.59	yeast, dried	4.98
		gelatin	1.78
Beverages			
cocoa powder	3.57		

Reference: Pennington, J. T. and Calloway, D. H. Copper content of foods. *Research* 63:143–153, 1973.

Of the trace elements tested, oral zinc plus manganese in a ratio of twenty to one will increase copper excretion via the urinary route. Molybdenum antagonizes copper absorption in sheep to the extent that naturally black sheep may grow depigmented wool when raised on feed with excess molybdenum. Data are not yet available for these three essential elements in Wilson's disease or even milder states of copper intoxication. Because this knowledge is lacking as regards man, patients are treated with more expensive and toxic chelating agents such as penicillamine, acetylcysteine and EDTA (ethylene diaminetetracetic acid).

These chelates are not specific for any one metal, but remove, via the urinary pathway, copper, zinc, lead, mercury and cadmium. This therapy is less than perfect since penicillamine also removes zinc from the body. Certainly, when penicillamine is used, the patient will lose his sense of taste if zinc and pyridoxine (B-6) are not given in adequate supply. The B-6 should be given at noon, while the penicillamine is given morning and night. Penicillamine will cause a two-hundredfold increase in urinary copper excretion. Patients sensitive to penicillin salts are usually also sensitive to penicillamine.

Avoiding Iron and Copper

Advertising campaigns promote iron-containing vitamins as a means of combating "iron-poor blood." As a result of this sales pitch, many vitamin-plus-mineral preparations predominantly contain iron and copper. We should attempt to rid the body of excess copper rather than look for new sources! In spite of this consideration, the large manufacturers of vitamin-and-mineral preparations see fit to follow the ancient Wisconsin patent which gives the dose of copper needed daily as 4 mg. Theragran-M and Geriplex have 2 mg of copper per capsule, while fifty other preparations in the *Physicians' Desk Reference* also contain copper. Many patients have zinc-poor tissues, and their fatigue may disappear when zinc plus vitamin B-6 is given as a dietary supplement.

References

Butt, E. M. et al. Trace metal patterns in disease states. *Amer. J. Clin. Pathol.* 30:474–497, 1958.

Gooch, R. Observations on puerperal insanity. *Med. Trans.* 6:263–324, 1820; *JAMA* 208:1697, 1969.

Lal, S.; Papeschi, R.; Duncan, R. J. S. and Sourkes, T. L. Effect of copper loading on various tissue enzymes and brain monoamines in the rat. *Toxicology and Applied Pharmacology* 28:395–405, 1974.

Linder, M. C. and Munro, H. N. *Enzyme* 15:111–113, 1973.

Peterson, H. and Swanson, A. G. *Arch. Intern. Med.* 113:877–880, 1974.

Pfeiffer, C. and Iliev, V. A study of zinc deficiency and copper excess in the schizophrenias. *Intern. Rev. of Neurobiol.* 141–165, 1972.

Roth, O. Myocardial infarct rate among young rises in U.S. *Int. Med. News*, 15 September 1974.

Schroeder, H. A. Essays in toxicology. 4:107–199, 1972.

Seelig, M. Proposed role of copper molybdenum interaction in iron-deficiency storage diseases. *Amer. J. Clin. Nutr.* 657–672, 1973.

Walker-Smith, J. and Bloomfield, J. Wilson's disease or chronic copper poisoning? *Arch. Diseases in Childhood* 48:476–478, 1973.

Copper Update 1978

Most patients at the Brain Bio Center are continually found to have high copper and low zinc levels. The biological antagonism between copper and zinc is common knowledge among animal nutritionists but is scarcely recognized by human nutritionists. We can learn much about this area simply by reading veterinary journals and studying trace element requirements for dogs and sheep. In one study, Bremner, et al. (1976) fed twelve-week-old lambs increasing doses of copper and determined what dose of zinc in the diet counteracted the copper poisoning produced by 30 mgm/kgm copper in the diet. He found that 420 mgm/kgm of zinc in the diet is needed to prevent the accumulation of copper in the liver. The ratio of zinc to copper is 420/30, or fourteen times more zinc than copper is needed. If we use this ratio as a guide, those multivitamins with minerals which give 2 mgm of copper per tablet should have 28 mgm of zinc per tablet to prevent accumulation of copper. *The Physicians' Desk Reference* gives popular preparations with 2 mgm of copper per tablet, but in these the zinc varies as follows: Theragran -M 1.5 mgm (as the sulfate), Myadec 1.5 mgm zinc, Geriplex 2 mgm of zinc sulfate, Optilets 500 zinc 1.5 mgm (as the sulfate) and Natalins Rx 15 mgm zinc similar to their Sustagen which has 2 mgm copper and 20 mg zinc per pound of powder. Only Natalins Rx and Sustagen of Mead-Johnson approach the ideal ratio of 1 copper to 14 zinc. We are assailed by copper in air, food and drinking water, but we must look hard to find the 15 mgm per day of zinc that is needed for the twenty or more reducing and transferring enzymes of the body. The copper is contained largely in enzymes that deal with the oxidative metabolism of the body.

Some Bedlington Terriers Have High Copper and Liver Damage

Owing to a genetic defect, the charming and playful Bedlington Terrier can develop high serum and tissue copper and liver damage. The afflicted dog is hyperactive as a pup and undergoes a personality change so that he will not frolic and play with other pups. Other symptoms are poor appetite, loss of hair, darkened skin and liver damage as shown by the elevation of SGPT and SGOT—liver enzymes. With 30 mgm of zinc A.M. and P.M. and 1 and 2 grams of vitamin C per day, the liver enzymes return to normal and the dog again becomes alert and playful—and stays that way with zinc and vitamin C therapy.

Patients Can Have Liver Damage from High Copper

When high copper or hypercupremia is mentioned as a diagnosis, the trained medical mind thinks *only* of Wilson's disease, a rare hereditary diesase that occurs in only 1 in 200,000 patients, usually children. In Clearwater, Florida, the water supply somehow became contaminated with copper, and twenty known adult cases of copper poisoning resulted. This was promptly labeled Wilson's disease. However, Clearwater, a suburb of St. Petersburg, has a population of less than 100,-000, and the odds are greatly against twenty adult cases of this rare disease occurring in a relatively small city.

Physicians must learn that copper can be a cause of liver disease. The whole matter boils down to "which is first, the chicken or the egg," since serum copper is always high in liver disease. From my intern days I recall the case of a thirteen-year-old farm girl who had fatal cirrhosis of the liver. Her ceruloplasm was normal, but the family history showed the installation of new copper plumbing (1937) and the use of copper kettles for cooking. The patient's serum and liver copper was high, but which was cause and which was effect? Perhaps the onset of puberty with the estrogens raising her copper intake made her more susceptible to copper poisoning.

Hard Water Protects Against Copper, Lead and Cadmium Poisoning

Scientists in the field of trace element research must be generalists, and as such, they cross pollinate many fields of research and know more and more about less and less—as do the specialists. Moreover, the discoveries and suggestions from their cross pollination require a decade or more for practical application in human preventive medicine. For example, the prevention of atherosclerosis by hard water is scientifically and epidemiologically sound. The level of calcium or magnesium in hard water is not enough to protect man. It may take a plumber, however, to graphically portray that hard water limes all pipes, whether copper or iron, and provides a protective coating against toxic elements in the pipes and joints of the drinking water supply. The plumber is called to replace the pipes when they lime shut. One environmentalist found the pH of his suburban town's drinking water to be 7.5. When the engineer in charge of the water supply was asked, he stated, that a high (alkaline) pH was needed to keep his water lines from leaking. He, therefore, added lime. In Oakland, California, and in reservoirs of other cities, the city biologists control the green algae in the water by the usual copper sulfate addition method. Crystalline $CuSo4$ (bluestone) is placed in a cloth sack behind a boat, which then travels around the lake or reservoir until the $CuSO4$ is dissolved. (The final product, the drinking water, is never analyzed for copper, although the U.S. Public Health Service sets upper limits of 1.0 ppm and the World Health Organization sets a limit of 0.05 ppm for copper in drinking water.)

High Serum Copper in Hypertension

Most of the hypertensive patients we see at the Brain Bio Center have low zinc and high serum copper. As zinc and vitamin C are given, both the lead and copper levels decrease. We cannot measure cadmium but that is probably also lowered with zinc and vitamin C therapy. The decrease in copper and lead is accompanied by a significant decrease in the elevated blood pressure—usually to a normal level. Blacks have a higher copper level than whites, and their hypertension is harder to treat with standard blood pressure lowering drugs. Black or skin tan pigment called melanin has a great affinity for copper, which might correlate with the higher copper and blood pressure in blacks. One might predict that elevated serum copper would be reduced by the tanning process of sunbathing. Maybe that is why sun worshipers get relaxed while their skin tans and becomes cancerous from the ultraviolet rays in sunlight.

Active Tuberculosis Elevates Copper and Lowers Zinc

Early studies postulated that schizophrenia and tuberculosis were somehow related, but with modern drugs to cure tuberculosis this connection has been disproven. Nonetheless, I still remember the schizoid behavior of many patients in the tuberculosis ward and the high incidence of tuberculosis among schizophrenics. Perhaps the low zinc and high copper engendered the schizophrenic behavior.

Copper Deficiency

A deficiency in copper rarely results from an inadequate diet. The element is ubiquitous; full-term infants are born with large stores in the liver which decrease with age.

Experimental copper deficiency is hard to induce in animals, even under the most restrictive conditions. All human cases of diet-induced deficiency have been related to prolonged intravenous feeding, long-term milk diets in infants and total malnourishment. Any of these factors may also lead to an iron-deficient anemia and other blood abnormalities. Copper aids in the absorption of iron in a non-specific way, in the same manner as cobalt and nickel. Patients with a copper deficiency have been more responsive to folic acid therapy than to copper supplementation.

Premature infants have many nutritional problems, among them copper deficiency. Both infants and adults on total intravenous feeding need to be carefully monitored for all nutritional problems, including copper deficiency.

The "Wort Won't Work" with Stainless Steel Alone

That copper is an essential trace element needed for normal cellular growth is evident from the statement of a brewmaster who came to us for preventive medical care. "We changed from copper to stainless steel throughout our brewery and found that the wort wouldn't work." By that he meant that the mixture of wheat, hops and malt that makes up the mix would not ferment into beer. The problem was not solved by adding copper salts to the wort but rather by the addition of a short section of copper piping. This piping supplied enough copper to make the wort work again. In this instance, the pure well water did not contain enough copper to sustain growth of the brewer's yeast.

DO COPPER IONS PROVIDE A NATURAL LIMITING REACTION TO ACUTE INFLAMMATION?

Numerous workers find that stress or infection is accompanied by a rise in serum copper and a decrease in serum zinc. Ward, et al. (1975) have studied the possible anti-inflammatory effect of gold, copper and zinc chlorides, wherein gold and copper are highly active and zinc is inactive. The white blood cell neutrophil chemotactic response can be 100 percent inhibited, but when washed the cells regain their normal responses. Gold salts are frequently used to reduce inflammation in rheumatoid arthritis. This suggests the role of heavy metals in a natural homeostatic mechanism in the body designed to limit the degree of inflammation. Severe inflammation in inappropriate places can be fatal—for example, brain edema or swelling in the voice box (larynx). Severe edema of an extremity can result in gangrene because of lack of blood supply.

Let us first summarize the studies that indicate that copper (or some copper compound) has an anti-inflammatory effect:

1. A copper-and-zinc-containing protein, *orgotein* (superoxide dismutase), ordinarily isolated from bovine liver is used in horses and other animals as a parenteral anti-inflammatory compound. A dose of only 5 mgm given subcutaneously will reduce acute inflammation within one hour.
2. The copper ion in small doses is anti-inflammatory.
3. At low dosage, copper ions enhance the anti-inflammatory effect of aspirin.
4. Copper decreases the gastric inflammation produced by aspirin and salicylates.
5. All simple anti-inflammatory drugs are potential chelators of bivalent metals such as copper, zinc, iron and calcium.
6. Estrogens raise serum copper, and estrogen therapy

may relieve arthritis in post-menopausal women. More women become arthritic after menopause.

7. Any stress, whether it be cancer, infection, pregnancy, joint disease or even athletic training, raises the serum copper level, which results in brain stimulation to the point of insomnia. This stimulation helps the athlete to set new records, but the insomnia further aggravates the condition of the patient who needs more rest.

8. Dr. M. W. Whitehouse, who has pioneered this thesis, also points to the patient's natural selection of foods high in copper, such as shellfish, nuts and cider vinegar. The persistent use of a copper bracelet is standard folklore and is a present-day custom to treat arthritis. Perhaps some skin absorption of copper occurs, and certainly the presence of sweaty fingers on a copper bracelet will result in transfer of copper from the bracelet to the mouth. If a copper compound is released during stress to limit the degree of inflammation, then another well-known observation might be explained. For instance, in cases of asphyxiation among adult males and females of the same age, the female lives longer and has less asphyxial damage. Because of estrogens, the female generally has higher copper levels than the male.

Superoxide Dismutase

Superoxide dismutase, an enzyme found in erythrocytes and liver cells, contains equimolar amounts of both zinc and copper. Low copper and low superoxide dismutase activity results in the accumulation of superoxide anion (O_2) in brain tissue. This anion is highly reactive and destroys adrenalin and noradrenaline.

The superoxide anion is the product of the oxidation of several substrates; xanthine catalyzed by xanthine oxidase proceeds by univalent reduction of O_2. Superoxide dismutase catalyzes the internal oxidation-reduction reaction of superoxide ion with hydrogen peroxide and O_2 as the products. In superoxide dismutase, at least one coordination position of the copper metal is left open, and alternating reduction and oxidation proceeds at this copper center. Zinc serves only as a bridge between different units of the enzyme. A deficiency in copper will result in reduced superoxide dismutase levels, accumulation of superoxides and a lower level of cathecholamines which are anti-inflammatory.

In a report by Dr. K. H. Falchuk of Boston on the action of the anti-flammatory hormone ACTH on zinc levels, with ACTH therapy the zinc serum levels, already low, fell significantly lower. Copper levels were not reported.

One should recall that the late Phillip Hench, a doctor at the Mayo Clinic, noted that jaundiced patients were relieved of their rheumatoid arthritis. This finding led to the discovery of cortisone, but we also know that in jaundiced patients the serum copper is high and the zinc is low.

The unique gastritis produced by the organic acids given for their anti-inflammatory effect may provide an important clue: simple inorganic acids and acetic acid are not corrosive to the gastric mucosa. These anti-inflammatory organic acids must remove a protecting chemical unit such as calcium (plus?) or copper (plus?) from the stomach lining. This new compound or complex should be present in the gastric or duodenal juices and might be recovered and analyzed.

DOES COPPER CHOP UP PYRIDOXINE (VITAMIN B-6)?

When the body is subject to stress, the serum zinc goes down and the copper goes up. This also occurs in women who use the birth control pill, with the result that all women on the pill should have extra zinc, B-6 and vitamin C. In liver disease the copper level is high and extra B-6 is chopped up rapidly as units of 100 mgm are given.

In acute heart disease the copper rises and the zinc falls, and here I can relate my own experience. Ordinarily I need 50 mgm of vitamin B-6 to have dream recall, but on vacation I dream too much and am awakened every two hours during the night with another vivid dream. Hence, I reduce my B-6 intake to 25 mgm per day, an intake that is still more than ten times the minimal daily requirement (MDR). Recently, during extreme cold weather in Princeton I had a minor heart attack which sent my copper up to 137 mcg percent (normally 90) and my zinc down to 110 mcg percent (normally 130). During my recovery I noted that I no longer had dream recall. The dose now needed for that normal phenomenon is 100 mgm daily or 50 times the MDR.

Summary

Many otherwise thoughtful nutritionists forget the meaning of the word *minimal* in MDR; recovery, convalescence or even active training for peak performance cannot be achieved on minimal doses of anything. For example, would minimal health or safety appeal to you? Minimal love in your life? Minimal orgasm with sex? We all want optimal health, safety, love and sexual experiences. We can attain these goals in spite of copper in our water, lead in our air and chemicals in our food if we take optimal doses of zinc, vitamin C and vitamin B-6.

References

Allen, R. Copper build-up traced to water. *The Tampa Tribune,* 28, August 1974.

Al-Rashid, R. A. and Spangler, J. Neonatal copper deficiency. *New England Journal of Medicine,* Medical Intelligence (Brief Recordings), 285:841–843, 7 October 1971.

Ashkenazi, A.; Levin, S.; Djaldetti, M.; Fishel, E. and Benvenisti, D. The syndrome of neonatal copper deficiency. *Pediatrics* 52(4):525–533, October 1973.

Beswick, P. H.; Hall, G. H.; Hook, A. J.; Little, K.; McBrien, D. C. H. and Lott, K. A. K. Copper toxicity: evidence for the conversion of cupric to cuprous copper in vivo under anaerobic conditions. *Chemical Biological Interactions* 14:347–356, 1976.

Bogden, J.; Lintz, D. I., Joselow, M. M.; Charles, J. and Salaki, J. S. Effect of pulmonary tuberculosis on blood concentrations of copper and zinc. *American Journal of Clinical Pathology* 67(3) March 1977.

Bremmer, I.; Young, B. W. and Mills, C. F. Protective effect of zinc supplementation against copper toxicosis in sheep. *British Journal of Nutrition* 36:551–561, 1976.

Burks, J.; Alfrey, A. C.; Huddlestone, J.; Norenberg, M. D. and Lewin, E. A fatal encephalopathy in chronic haemodialysis patients. *The Lancet*, 10 April 1976, pp. 764–768.

Copper metabolism in patients with liver disease. *Nutrition Reviews* 35(6):136–138, June 1977.

Drink kept in brass pot causes copper poisoning. *Medical Tribune Report*, Atlanta, 19 March 1975.

Falchuk, K. H. Effect of acute disease and ACTH on serum zinc proteins. *New England Journal of Medicine* 296(20):1129–1134, 1977.

Fee, J. A. and Ward, R. L. Evidence for a coordination position available to solute molecules on one of the metals at the active center of reduced bovine superoxide dismutase. *Biochemical and Biophysical Research Communications* 71(2):427–437, 1976.

Goette, D. K. and Odom, R. B. Alopecia in crash dieters. *JAMA* 235(24):2622–2623, 14 June 1976.

Graham, G. G. and Cordano, A. Copper depletion and deficiency in the malnourished infant. *Johns Hopkins Medical Journal* 124(3):139–150, March 1969.

Hambidge, M. K. The role of zinc and other trace metals in pediatric nutrition and health. *Pediatric Clinics of North America* 24(1):95–106, February 1977.

Haralambie, G.; Keul, J. and Theumert, F. Protein-, Eisen- und Kupfer-Veränderungen im serum bei Schwimmern vor und nach Höhentraining. *European Journal of Applied Physiology* 35:21–31, 1976.

Henderson, B. M. and Winterfield, R. W. Acute copper

toxicosis in the Canada goose. *Avian Diseases* (Case Report) 19(2):385–387, April–June 1975.

Karpel, J. T. and Peden, V. H. Copper deficiency in long-term parenteral nutrition. *Journal of Pediatrics* 80(1):32–36, January 1972.

Lawler, M. R. and Jelenc, M. A. Recipes for low-copper diets. *Journal of the American Dietetic Association* 57(5):420–422, November 1970.

Mylrea, P. J. and Byrne, D. T. An outbreak of acute copper poisoning in calves. *Australian Veterinary Journal* 50:169, April 1974.

O'Dell, B. L. *Biochemistry and physiology of copper*, pp. 404–407.

O'Dell, B. L.; Smith, R. M. and King, R. A. Effect of copper status on brain neurotransmitter metabolism in the lamb. *Journal of Neurochemistry* 26:451–455, 1976.

Potts, A. M. and Au, C. P. The affinity of melanin for inorganic ions. *Experimental Eye Research* 22:487–491, 1976.

Ritland, S.; Steinnes, E. and Skrede, S. Hepatic copper content, urinary copper excretion, and serum ceruloplasmin in liver disease. *Scandinavian Journal of Gastroenterology* 12:81–88, 1977.

Robitaille, G. A.; Piscatelli, R. L.; Majeski, E. J. and Gelehrter, T. D. Hemolytic anemia in Wilson's disease. A report of three cases with transient increase in hemoglobin A2. *JAMA* 237(22):2402–2403, 30 May 1977.

Sass-Kortsak, A. Wilson's disease, a treatable liver disease in children. *Pediatric Clinics of North America* 22(4):963–984, November 1975.

Suttle, N. F. and Angus, K. W. Experimental copper deficiency in the calf. *Journal of Comparative Pathology* 86:595–608, 1976.

Vaisrub, S. Ravages of copper in early Wilson's disease. *JAMA* 237(22):2413, 30 May 1977.

Vilter, R. W.; Bozian, R. C.; Hess, E. V.; Zellner, D. C. and Petering, H. G. Manifestations of copper deficiency in a patient with systemic sclerosis on intravenous hyperalimentation. *New England Journal of Medicine* 291:188–191, 25 July 1974.

Walsh, F. M.; Crosson, F. J.; Bayley, M.; McReynolds, J. and Pearson, B. J. Acute copper intoxication. *American Journal of Disease of Children* 131:149–151, 1977.

Ward, P. A.; Goldschmidt, P. and Greener, N. D. Suppressive effects of metal salts on leukocyte and fibroblastic function. *Journal of the Reticuloendothilial Society* 18(5):315–321, 1975.

Whitehouse, M. W. Ambivalent role of copper in inflammatory disorders. *Agents and Actions* 6:201–206, 1976.

Ylostalo, P. and Ylikorkala, O. Hepatosis of pregnancy, a clinical study of 107 patients. *Annales Chirurgiae et Gynaecologiae Fenniae* 64:128–134, 1975.

CHAPTER 20

Bismuth:
The Fifth [Column]
Heavy Metal

In addition to mercury, lead, cadmium, and copper, another metal has been discovered to be a cause of mental symptoms. Bismuth is a heavy metal which has no known natural function in man, animals or plants. Primarily in Australia, bismuth subgallate is prescribed to be taken orally, in a powdered form. Bismuth has been used in the past for treating syphilis, and mental symptoms such as are now described were not seen with overdosage.

Patients who have undergone a colostomy (an operation in which an artificial opening is formed in the abdominal wall) are frequently given bismuth salts in order to reduce fecal odor and regulate elimination. Dr. James F. Robertson of Australia has reported cases of bismuth intoxication which could erroneously be diagnosed as mental illness. The use of bismuth subgallate produced a staggering gait, difficulty in memory recall, tremor, disturbances of vision and hearing, and difficulty in estimating time and distance. In some cases, auditory and visual hallucinations occurred. The symptoms disappeared when the salt of bismuth was discontinued.

Other preparations which contain bismuth are certain rectal suppositories for the relief of pain and discomfort, and some antidiarrhea medicines containing bismuth, pectin and paragoric. In light of the potential mental effects, we advise avoidance of repeated oral use of products which contain bismuth in any form. "Pepto-Bismol" is the most advertised product.

Bismuth and Zinc

The time course of return of memory and relief of other symptoms would suggest that bismuth may interfere with the absorption of zinc from the small intestine. If bismuth were lodged in the brain, the patient would need extensive chelation therapy to reverse the intoxication. In Dr. Robertson's experience, the symptoms decreased when the dose of bismuth was reduced. The gallic acid molecule is similar to the phytic acid molecule, so that the repeated use of bismuth subgallate could result in zinc deficiency. If bismuth subgallate produces zinc deficiency, this can be proven by blood serum analysis for zinc. Zinc deficiency would produce the reversible intoxication which is described in the following case history from Australia.

Patient Writes

Dear Mr. A.,

Further to our phone conversation of today I outline the main things that I experienced when I nearly died in Prince Henry's hospital and the symptoms that built up on (and in) me during the four years that passed after my colostomy operation under Mr. Hughes till I was carried in a complete coma into Prince Henry's.

Mr. Hughes told me my operation was eminently successful and that in five weeks I should be normal and back at work. I felt lousy at that time and was quite unable to work. No other adjective describes my feeling.

I first noticed a peculiar sensation in the tips of the fingers and toes and a kind of perpetual neuritis. I put it down to the drugs in hospital. I had then been on bismuth subgallate for about a month when these symptoms started.

After six months still feeling rotten I went back to work at T.P.N.G. thinking that would be therapeutic.

To my dismay I found that the control of my heat in my body was in disarray. I was overhot and sweated profusely or overcold and clammy. It was most distressing after 40 years normal life in the tropics.

I stuck at things for 12 months in T.P.N.G. and then resigned and returned hoping that the cold climate and less onerous life would cure me.

I took up work about the home, repair and alteration, little mental work and lived simply and healthy. But there was no real improvement. My mental powers deteriorated, memory, reading and writing ability and sight. I twitched all over especially at night. My breathing started to be affected, shortness of breath at times and peculiar momentary breath in the inhaling process when my lungs were about half full.

I found my manual work increasingly difficult over three years. I finally had to stop as I could not hold a tool steady. I could not do my buttons or hold a tea cup steady and level except with major concentration. I lost my balance and was continually falling over. This so degenerated that I would fall over twitching and sight all went out of order. My feet swelled so I had to get large shoes.

I lost my ability to laugh or smile. I could not work the muscles of my face. I also became rather moon faced. I could not keep the car off the gravel edge of the road and within the white lines so I gave up driving. I completely lost my sense of direction and geography of Melbourne.

I became a great sufferer from insomnia. I twitched so much and also could not lie still in bed but had to turn from side to side every minute or so. I was put on various drugs but none really helped. I forgot their names, but each drug's effect wore off fairly soon and I had to be given another. In the day time however I could not keep awake. I used to fall into a so-called sleep (though it was not that) even when talking to friends. My wife tried everything to keep me awake in the day time so I might sleep at night. But it did nothing to help me sleep normally. Waking from this "sleep" in the day time was a horrid experience. One seemed to be climbing up and out of a deep unconsciousness. I felt that one day I just would not climb out! I'd be dead. I dreaded each day time as I could not do anything up about the house or rest in bed at night. Too I dreaded the nights also. I was very disorientated and mentally could not remember things and did strange things at times and my wife had to watch me very carefully.

I had a relapse and into Repat., where they cut my intestine back about 4″ and this helped with handling my equipment and comfort. However my general condition which was now diagnosed as a nervous one and possibly of psychological origin did not improve. Finally after 5½ years I fell over in the garden in a coma and was carried into Prince Henry's Hospital. (By the way I had become incontinent.) I was in P.H. about six weeks, violent and strapped to my bed, with a surround to keep me in bed. I can remember patches of the awful nightmares which took hold of me. The doctors told my wife that all the tests made showed that my brain was dying rapidly though my body was relatively strong. After three or four weeks of this I grew quieter and one afternoon I opened my eyes suddenly and saw my wife at my bedside and spoke rationally with and to her. She hurried away and told the doctor and he came and did various simple brain tests and then took my wife away and told her they would have to reassess my case as I appeared to have suddenly become rational. Now the only thing in my treatment that had changed in Prince Henry's was that I had not had any bismuth subgallate. All the other drugs were carried on when they could get them into me. I think I was taking three powerful drugs all the time. I forgot their names.

P.H. decided to keep me on longer as I was rational (fairly) instead of sending me to a nursing home to slowly die. After a fortnight further I went out to Wattle Glen Private Hospital and had 12 weeks there with marvellous nursing. They got me on my feet and restored my balance partly. I was beginning to smile again though somewhat weakly.

I returned home not normal but well enough not to be intolerable burden. Over two years all my symptoms have disappeared slowly. I can work again, breathe normally, don't twitch, think again, enjoy books, T.V., my technical skills returned normally and mentally (I have very comprehensive technical training).

My sense of direction and geography returned and my driving skill. I wear my old size shoes again. My sight has returned to normal and I wear my old glasses. This return to health was very slow and gradual but I never looked back. Balance is now quite okay. When I got to the dentist he found my teeth *heavily stained yellow* (with bismuth subgallate?) and under very bad decay. Previously I had excellent teeth. I am constantly in this man's hands for repairs.

I had a peculiar ache in my arms as though my biceps were affected. My lungs (?) or there abouts also ached in different areas. These aches have all gone after two years at home.

Well I think that is enough. I dislike writing about it because it is all about "me" and ego certainly is the very devil. But I only write this thinking it may help somebody. My family doctor told his wife who told my wife he had reported this matter of bismuth subgallate to the proper authorities and I hope he has. I feel it is a slow and insidious poison to those persons who are allergic to it. I also feel that some folk on it after a colostomy though not reacting as we did never the less may be suffering poor health and blaming their colostomy for this. I only use charcoal tablets now and don't take any other drugs except odd vitamins. I found Vitamin C helps the improvement of my salivary system and dry mouth which seems to be one of the few disabilities I still have.

P.S. I call to mind some drugs, Stelazine, Seconal, Vallium and one they take for epilepsy—I forgot that one—Tryptanol I believe was another. But I don't think these caused my troubles as my down hill drive started after my colostomy operation the drugs came much later and I had no withdrawal symptoms as these were all gradually taken away.

I hope you can decipher this and get out of it all the tones of what I say. My writing is never good and I am too lazy to peck away at my typewriter.

                              With kind regards, A.B.
P.P.S. I should add that I am firmly convinced I am alive today only by the intervention of the Lord in and through my circumstances.

References

Robertson, J. F. Mental illness or metal illness? Bismuth subgallate. *Med. J. of Australia* 1:887–888, 1974.

Bismuth Update 1978

Bismuth poisoning has now been reported from regions all over the world, including Germany (two cases), Australia (twenty-nine) and France (about thirty). Since the Australians were first to discover modern bismuth poisoning, they have discovered more cases. In the United States patients with bismuth poisoning may go unrecognized.

Bismuth as the subsalicylate is present in Peptobismol, an over-the-counter remedy for stomach upset and diarrhea. While the use of bismuth salts for short periods (four weeks) has proved helpful in healing duodenal and gastric ulcers, prolonged use results in poisoning. Bismuth, like mercury, is also a component of many commercially available cosmetics that are used to lighten skin blemishes. These cosmetics are available without prescription.

Bismuth salts are frequently ingested after a colostomy (a fourth teaspoon bismuth subgallate after each meal) to control fecal odor and regulate the bowels. The first symptoms in a few weeks are mental confusion, slurring of speech, and clumsiness; later, arthropathies (joint problems) and myoclonus (muscle twitches and spasms) occur. Patients have disturbed oxidative cerebral metabolism, increased lactate production and decreased oxygen and glucose consumption. Prolonged or unrecognized poisoning results in loss of memory, difficulty in motion and eventually coma. It takes from five to twelve weeks for the symptoms to recede when exposure to bismuth is stopped. Damage does not seem to be permanent, for all patients recovered. Injections of calcium and magnesium may result in a more rapid recovery. Zinc at an oral dose of 30 mgm A.M. and P.M. should be tried. While poisoned with bismuth, a woman gave birth to two children, both of whom were apparently normal.

Blood bismuth levels in a patient suffering from bismuth poisoning, who recovered slowly after ingestion of salts was stopped, were as follows:

1/28/75—900 ug/liter	
2/ 1/75—380 ug/liter	With acute symptoms, blood
2/11/75—100 ug/liter	bismuth levels range from
2/24/75— 75 ug/liter	210 ug/liter to 1470 ug/liter.
3/ 3/75— 40 ug/liter	

Lymphocytes occurred in the cerebral spinal fluid up to 100 cells per cu mm in this patient.

Poisoning has been reported from prolonged use of several bismuth salts, i.e., the subgallate, subnitrate and subcarbonate (in order of decreasing toxicity). The mode of toxicity is unknown, but several theories have been proposed: bismuth metylation by the body to a more toxic form, or chelation of zinc by the acid of the salt. Neither of these theories has been verified. It seems certain that the poisoning is the result of bismuth being absorbed slowly over a span of several months or years. Stopping the ingestion of bismuth salts results in a rapid decrease in blood level and slow relief of symptoms. More cases of bismuth poisoning will be found if we learn to look for it.

References

Allain, P.; Alquier, P.; and Dumont, A. M. Etude expérimentale de l'elimination du bismuth per hemodialyse. *Thĕrapie* 31: 703–706, 1976.

Boudouresques, J.; Khalil, R.; Cherif, A. A. and Boudouresques, G. Encephalopathies au bismuth. *La Nouvelle Presse Medicale*, 13 September 1975.

Buge, A.; Hubault, A. and Rancorel, G. Les arthropathies de l'intoxication par le bismuth. *Revue du Rhumatisme* 42(12):721–729, 1975.

Escourolle, R.; Bourdon, R.; Galli, A.; Galle, P.; Jaudon,

M. C.; Hauw, J. J. and Gray, F. Neuropathological and toxicological study of twelve cases of bismuth encephalopathy. *Rev. Neurol.* 133(3):153–165, 1977.

Kruger, G.; Thomas, D. J.; Weinhardt, F. and Hpyer, S. Disturbed oxidative metabolism in organic brain syndrome caused by bismuth skin creams. *The Lancet* 9/4:485–497, 1976.

Lechat, P.; Palliere, M.; Gernez, G.; Dechy, H. and Letterton, N. Repartition comparée du bismuth dans l'organisme du rat aprés administration orale répétée de differents sels. *Annal Pharmaceutiqeus Francaises* 34(5–6):179–182, 1976.

Moshal, M. G. A bismuth peptide complex in the treatment of duodenal ulceration. *S. Afr. Med. J.* 49:1157–1159, 1975.

Scobie, B. A. Successful bismuth (De-Nol) therapy for gastric ulcer. *New Zealand Med. J.* 84:192–193, 1976.

CHAPTER 21

Summary

Special Brain Bio Center Vitamin and Mineral Supplements

THE DIET SHOULD CONTAIN as much as possible of the following foods: whole grains and whole grain bread, fresh or dried fruits, wheat germ, sprouted seeds, legumes (such as lentils, peas and beans), nuts, cheese, eggs, milk, brewer's yeast, skimmed milk powder, sea food, poultry, organ meats and lean meats. In addition, safflower oil should be taken at the level of at least 1 tablespoon daily. The oil can be mixed with wheat germ and used as the morning cereal with milk and fruit.

The Brain Bio Center treats both "normal people" and patients from a metabolic-nutritional viewpoint. The family physician can be in charge of normal nutrition, and even simple vitamin preparations, but should not prescribe commercial *vitamins plus minerals*. These are loaded with copper which our whole population gains in excess from copper plumbing. We recommend distilled or bottled water if the house water supply is high in copper. Brass activated-carbon filters actually may add more copper to the drinking water.

The special preparations most frequently needed according to age are:

INFANTS

Pyri-Zinc
  In
Dropping
Bottles

Willner Chemists
330 Lexington Avenue
New York City, N.Y. 10016

Contains

100 mgm B-6/ml
50 mgm zinc/ml as
the gluconate

B-6 and zinc drops

Bronson Pharmaceuticals
4526 Rinetti Lane
La Canada, Calif. 91011

Contains

175 mgm B-6/ml
12.5 mgm zinc/ml as
the gluconate

For newborn infants, the starting dose may be as low
as 1 drop per day.

CHILDREN

The zinc and B-6 liquid preparations listed above can
also be used in children but at a correspondingly
greater dosage. Pleasant dream recall is normal, and
B-6 will cause pleasant dreams which can be recalled
each morning. White spotted nails are a sign of zinc
deficiency, and zinc gluconate 15 mgm A.M. and P.M.
should be given; zinc and vitamin C, 1 to 2 grams per
day, may be needed to lower the lead level of children
who live along our arterial highways (lead pollution
from auto exhaust).

TEEN-AGERS

The hormones at puberty make great demands for adequate mineral intake which are *not met by jiffy foods*
or standard vitamins plus minerals (too high in cop-

per). Acne, amenorrhea and microphallus can result from zinc deficiency.

Teen-agers need

Vitamin C	2.0 gms/day
B-6	Enough for dream recall

Ziman Fortified capsules—a source of zinc and manganese	Willner Chemists 330 Lexington Avenue New York City, N.Y. 10016
Vicon Plus capsules **Iodized Salt or Kelp tablet** daily	Meyer Laboratories Ft. Lauderdale, Fla. 33309

Girls who scarcely eat meat should have one Mol-Iron tablet each day. This provides iron and the essential trace element molybdenum which may help to control excess bone growth at puberty.

ADULTS

Adults, in addition to natural foods, usually need zinc and manganese with vitamin C.

Vicon Plus or Ziman Fortified	1 capsule per day
Copper-free drinking water	

The manganese in Vicon Plus or Ziman Fortified may elevate blood pressure, in which case zinc alone should be taken each day.

Vicon-C or Zimag C **or zinc gluconate**	15 to 30 mgm A.M. and P.M.
Brewer's yeast	3 tablets A.M. and P.M. (for chromium containing glucose tolerance factor)

Vitamin C	2 gm/day
Safflower oil	1 tablespoon
Dolomite (if not drinking milk)	
Vitamin A	25,000 u daily
Vitamin E	400 u daily

GERIATRIC PATIENTS

In addition to natural foods, vitamin C, zinc, B-6, brewer's yeast, safflower oil and copper-free drinking water, senior citizens have special needs. These are:

Calcium dolomite	2 tablets A.M. and P.M.
Magnesium oxide	2 of 300 mgm A.M. and P.M.
Vitamin A	25,000 u daily
Vitamin E	400 u daily
Vitamin B-12	100 mcg/day
Folic acid	0.4 mgm/day
Inositol	A.M. and P.M.
Lecithin	A.M. and P.M.

CONCLUSION

We hope that this book on Minerals (M), Micro-Nutrients (Mn) and Heavy Metals (HM) will alert physicians, patients, parents and nurses to the need for the natural M and Mn and the dire effects on the human body of HM, the heavy metals. M and Mn can be out of balance; HM can be an unsuspected intruder which upsets the balance between M and Mn in the body.

Obviously the public, the teachers and the medical profession must be educated to understand that minerals and micronutrients can be essential to normal vitality. Food in its natural state contains more M and Mn than processed foods and should be given preference. But natural foods must be carefully guarded against the HM impurities.

INDEX

A

Acanthosis, zinc deficiency and, 11

Acne, 50

Acrodermatitis enteropathica (AE), 50, 53, 54

Adolescent(s): acne of, 50; hypogonadism and zinc deficiency, 6, 17, 44-45; iron deficiency in, 58; male growth lag, 16-17; male impotence, 12; masturbation and zinc loss, 45-46; recommended dietary supplements, 235; sexual immaturity and zinc deficiency, 6, 11-12, 17, 44-45, 50

Adults: chronic zinc deficiency effects, 17; recommended dietary supplements, 235-236

Aluminum, 153-155, 156-160; absorption and serum phosphorus, 159; body distribution, 153-154, 156; in drinking water, 154, 156, 159-160; brain and, 154-155, 156-157, 158, 159; pre-senile dementia and, 158, 159; serum phosphorus and, 153, 157; skin and, 154, 157; toxicity, 156-157, 159, 160

Alzheimer's disease, 158, 159

Anemia: cobalt for, 138-139; copper-molybdenum in, 203; defined, 59; high tin levels in, 134; irondeficiency related to pyridoxinedeficiency, 58, 60; nickel and, 152; pernicious, 60; phosphate and, 100; symptoms, 59-60; therapy of, 63-64; zinc and, 11

Antacids: encephalopathy and, 156-157; magnesium and, 105; serum phosphate and, 153, 157

Arteriosclerosis: chromium and, 131; magnesium and, 103, 105, 106

Arthritis, histidine for, 9; *See also* Rheumatoid arthritis

Ascorbic acid. *See* Vitamin C

Atherosclerosis: hard water and, 215; manganese and, 67

Autism, 53; copper and, 179, 205; lead and, 179, 205; mercury and, 205; zinc supplements in, 53

B

Birth defects: fluoridation of water and, 144; metals in drinking water and, 160; zinc deficiency and, 14-15

Bismuth, 225-231; intoxication, 225, 226, 230-231; mental illness and, 225, 230; use of preparations with, 225-226, 230; zinc absorption and, 226-229

Blood: coagulation, 72, 90, 93; garlic and, 82; selenium in, 85, 87-88

Blood pressure: calcium excess in hypertension, 216; chromium deficiency and, 131; garlic and, 82; nickel and adrenalin action on, 149; sodium and potassium and, 112-113; zinc-manganese supplements and, 25

Bone(s): calcium and, 90-91, 93, 97; fluoride and, 140, 142, 143, 145; magnesium and calcium mobilization from, 105-106; phosphate and, 154; magnesium in neoplasms, 102-103

Brain: aluminum and, 154-155, 156-157, 158, 159; bismuth and, 225, 230; copper in, 9, 163, 200, 202; histamine as neurotransmitter, 10; iron in, 9, 163; lead in, 163, 167; magnesium in, 9, 103; manganese and, 67-68, 71-72; mercury in, 173; zinc in, 9, 10-11, 42, 163

Brewer's yeast, glucose tolerance factor and, 127, 129, 132

Burns, zinc depletion in, 13, 17

C

Cadmium: calcium metabolism and, 174; infertility and, 43; in plated

237